Nail Therapies

Nail Therapies
Current Clinical Practice

Edited by

Robert Baran MD
Honorary Professor
University of Franche-Comté
Nail Disease Center
Cannes, France

Dimitris Rigopoulos MD, PhD
Professor of Dermatology-Venereology
School of Health Sciences
National and Kapodistrian University of Athens
Athens, Greece

Chander Grover MD, DNB, MNAMS
Professor of Dermatology
University College of Medical Sciences and GTB Hospital
Delhi, India

Eckart Haneke MD
Dermatology Practice Dermaticum, Freiburg, Germany
Centro de Dermatología Epidermis, Instituto CUF, Porto, Portugal
Kliniek voor Huidziekten, Universitair Ziekenhuis, Ghent, Belgium
and
Department of Dermatology
Inselspital, University of Bern
Bern, Switzerland

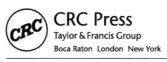

CRC Press
Taylor & Francis Group
Boca Raton London New York

CRC Press is an imprint of the
Taylor & Francis Group, an **informa** business

First edition published 2021
by CRC Press
6000 Broken Sound Parkway NW, Suite 300, Boca Raton, FL 33487-2742

and by CRC Press
2 Park Square, Milton Park, Abingdon, Oxon, OX14 4RN

© 2021 Taylor & Francis Group, LLC

CRC Press is an imprint of Taylor & Francis Group, LLC

Library of Congress Cataloging-in-Publication Data
Names: Baran, R. (Robert) editor. | Rigopoulos, Dimitris, editor. | Grover, Chander, editor. | Haneke, Eckart, editor.
Title: Nail therapies : current clinical practice / edited by Robert Baran, MD, Honorary Professor, University of Franche-Comté, Nail Disease Center, Cannes, France, Dimitris Rigopoulos, MD, PhD, Professor of Dermatology-Venereology, School of Health Sciences, National and Kapodistrian University of Athens, Greece, Chander Grover, MD, DNB, MNAMS, Professor of Dermatology, University College of Medical Sciences and GTB Hospital, Delhi, India, Eckart Haneke, MD, Department of Dermatology, Inselspital, University of Bern, Switzerland, Dermatology Practice Dermaticum, Freiburg, Germany, Centro de Dermatología Epidermis, Instituto CUF, Porto, Portugal Kliniek voor Huidziekten, Universitair Ziekenhuis, Ghent, Belgium.
Description: Second edition. | Boca Raton : CRC Press, 2021. | Summary: "A succinct guide to treatment options, both medical and surgical, for both disorders and injuries of the nail"--Provided by publisher.
Identifiers: LCCN 2020049409 (print) | LCCN 2020049410 (ebook) | ISBN 9780367334796 (hardback) | ISBN 9780367334789 (paperback) | ISBN 9781003159117 (ebook)
Subjects: LCSH: Nails (Anatomy) | Diagnosis, Differential. | Nails (Anatomy)--Diseases.
Classification: LCC RL94 .N35 2021 (print) | LCC RL94 (ebook) | DDC 611/.78--dc23
LC record available at https://lccn.loc.gov/2020049409
LC ebook record available at https://lccn.loc.gov/2020049410

ISBN: 978-0-367-33479-6 (hbk)
ISBN: 978-0-367-33478-9 (pbk)
ISBN: 978-1-003-15911-7 (ebk)

Typeset in Times
by MPS Limited, Dehardun

Contents

Preface

The success of the first edition of *Nail Therapies*, which has now been published in several other languages, encouraged us to broaden the field we had originally chosen. COVID-19 and the subsequent lockdown was the spark which kindled our flame. We consequently surrounded ourselves with undisputed competent colleagues, in order to reach out to readers eager for knowledge in this specialty topic that is still comparatively unknown — the Nail Apparatus.

We would like this edition to be both practical and useful for as long as possible, even if, sooner or later, it will inevitably be necessary to update the contents as therapeutics advance.

The comments and opinions of readers are very important to us and we therefore sincerely thank them in advance for their participation in the therapeutic progress that will contribute to and inspire our own Nail Appendage.

Robert Baran
Dimitris Rigopoulos
Chander Grover
Eckart Haneke

Contributors

Richard Encaoua, Dermatologie-oncologie, Centre médical des Batignolles, Paris, France

Geetali Kharghoria, Department of Dermatology and Venereology, All India Institute of Medical Sciences, New Delhi, India

Shari R. Lipner, Department of Dermatology, Weill Cornell Medicine, New York, New York, USA

Annie Pillet, Pillet Hand Prostheses, Paris, France

Jose W. Ricardo, Department of Dermatology, Weill Cornell Medicine, New York, New York, USA

1

Anatomy and physiology of the nail unit

Dimitris Rigopoulos

The nail plate is the permanent product of the nail matrix. Its normal appearance and growth depend on the integrity of several components such as the tissues surrounding the nail, or perionychium, the bony phalanx that contribute to the nail apparatus or nail unit (Figure 1.1).

The nail is a semi-hard horny plate covering the dorsal aspect of the tip of the digit. The nail is inserted proximally in an invagination practically parallel to the upper surface of the skin and laterally in the lateral nail grooves. This pocket-like invagination has a roof, the proximal nail fold, and a floor, the matrix from which the nail is derived.

The matrix extends approximately 6 mm under the proximal nail fold, and its distal portion is only visible as the white semi-circular lunula. The general shape of the matrix is a crescent concave in its posteroinferior portion. The lateral horns of this crescent are more developed in the great toe and located at the coronal plane of the bone. The ventral aspect of the proximal nail fold encompasses both a lower portion, the matrix, and an upper portion (roughly three-quarters of its length) called the eponychium.

The germinal matrix forms the bulk of the nail plate. The proximal element forms the superficial third of the nail, whereas the distal element covers its inferior by two-thirds.

The ventral surface of the proximal nail fold adheres closely to the nail for a short distance and forms a gradually desquamating tissue, the cuticle, made of the stratum corneum of both the dorsal and the ventral side of the proximal nail fold. The cuticle seals and, therefore, protects the ungual cul-de-sac from harmful environmental agents.

The nail plate is bordered by the proximal nail fold, which is continuous with the similarly structured lateral nail fold on each side. The nail bed extends from the lunula to the hyponychium. It presents with parallel longitudinal rete ridges.

The nail bed, in contrast to the matrix, has a firm attachment to the nail plate. Therefore, its avulsion produces a denudation of the nail bed. Colorless but translucent, the highly vascular connective tissue containing glomus organs transmits a pink color through the nail.

Distally, adjacent to the nail bed, the hyponychium, an extension of the volar epidermis under the nail plate, marks the point at which the nail separates from the underlying tissue.

The distal nail groove, which is convex anteriorly, separates the hyponychium from the fingertip.

Circulation of the nail apparatus is supplied by two digital arteries that course along the digits and send out branches to the distal and proximal arches.

The sensory nerves to the dorsum of the distal phalanx of the three middle fingers are derived from fine oblique dorsal branches of the volar collateral nerves. Longitudinal branches of the dorsal collateral nerves supply the terminal phalanx of the fifth digit and the thumb.

Among its multiple functions, the nail provides counterpressure for the pulp that is essential to the tactile sensation involving the fingers and for the prevention of distal wall tissue produced after nail loss of the great toenail.

The nail is a musculoskeletal appendage as a part of a functional unit that is comprised of the distal bony phalanx and several structures of the distal interphalangeal joint extensor tendon fibers and the

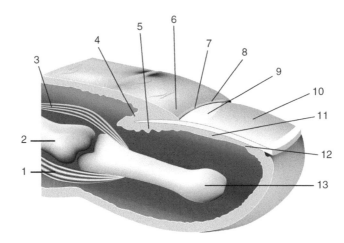

FIGURE 1.1   Anatomy of the nail apparatus: 1. flexor tendon; 2. middle phalanx; 3. extensor tendon; 4. eponychium; 5. nail matrix; 6. proximal nail fold; 7. cuticle; 8. lateral nail fold; 9. lunula; 10. nail plate; 11. nail bed; 12. hyponychium; 13. terminal phalanx.

collateral ligaments. All these form the enthesis (Figure 1.2). This organ is the bony insertion point of the ligaments, the tendons, and the articular capsules. It is composed of both

- Soft tissue (ligaments, tendons, and their fibrocartilages)
- Hard tissue (calcified fibrocartilage, the immediately adjacent bone of the underlying trabecular network)

Histological images confirm the link between the different structures.

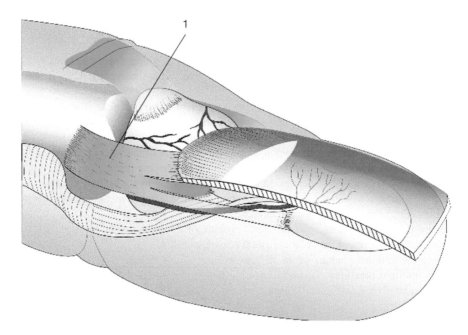

FIGURE 1.2   Entheses of the nail apparatus with (1) dorsal expansion of the lateral ligament at the distal interphalangeal joint (Guerro's ligament).

Histology permits recognition of the nail matrix and nail bed that have no granular layer, in contrast to the upper ventral aspect of the proximal nail fold called eponychium and the hyponychium.

The hard keratin of the nail lies perpendicularly to the nail growth axis and parallel to the surface of the nail plate.

Fingernails grow continuously on an average of 0.1 mm per day (3 mm per month). Toenails form over a period of 12–18 months.

The nail unit is in some respects comparable to a hair follicle sectioned longitudinally and laid on its side. The epithelial components of hair follicle and nail apparatus are differentiated epidermal structures that may be involved jointly in several ways, such as lichen planus and alopecia areata.

- Only the nail matrix produces the nail plate.
- No bone, no nail.
- Knowledge of growth rate is often helpful in establishing the disease onset.
- Entheses play an important role in nail anatomy.

FURTHER READING

De Berker DAD, André J., Baran R. (2007) Nail biology and nail science. *Int J Cosm Sci*; 29: 241–275.
McGonagle D., Tan A. L., Benjamin M. (2008) The biomechanical link between skin and joint disease in psoriasis and psoriatic arthritis: what every dermatologist needs to know. *Ann Rheum Dis*; 67: 1–9.
Morgan A. M., Baran R., Haneke E. (2001) Anatomy of the nail unit in relation to the distal digit. In Krull E. A., Zook E. G., Baran R., Haneke E. (eds). *Nails Surgery. A Text Atlas*. Lippincott William Wilkins, Philadelphia PA, 1–28.

2

Psoriasis

Dimitris Rigopoulos

Psoriasis is presented in various forms involving different parts of the nail unit, as shown in Table 2.1.

Pits

These are the commonest signs of psoriasis. They are mainly seen on fingernails. Nail disease most typically affects the dominant hand thumbnail and then the other nails that are most associated with hand function. Incidence of fingernail pitting increases with the total duration and severity of the disease. They are deeper than those in alopecia areata and also more numerous, and they can be transient or in some cases, long lasting. The presence of more than 20 pits suggests a psoriatic cause of the nail dystrophy, while more than 60 pits per person are unlikely to be found in the absence of psoriasis. There is no sex predilection while concerning age; patients over 40 years are affected twice as often as those under 20 years. It is also notable that several pits can result in trachyonychia-like appearance of the nails. When the psoriatic lesion affects a wider area of the nail matrix, transverse grooves (onychomadesis) are formed in the same way as pits. They are due to involvement of the proximal part of the nail matrix, resulting in abnormal cornification and presence of parakeratotic corneocytes in the nail plate. These cells, as they are loosely attached, drop out, leaving punctuate depressions on the nail plate (resembling a thimble), which correspond to the pits (Figure 2.1). The parakeratotic cells that remain are visible like scales within the pits.

Subungual Hyperkeratosis

This is due to the inflammation of the hyponychium and the distal nail bed and the hyperplasia of the epidermis. The keratin layer is trapped, in a way, under the surface of the nail plate (Figure 2.2). Subungual hyperkeratosis affects the toenails more frequently than the fingernails. Subungual hyperkeratosis in psoriasis is usually silvery white due to the air that enters the elevated distal end of the nail plate. This color may change if there is a secondary infection.

Oil-Drop Sign (Salmon Patch)

This is a color change (yellow or salmon pink) of the nail plate, characteristic of the disease. It is due to the trapping of neutrophils under the surface of the nail plate. It is located centrally or by the onycholytic area (Figure 2.3). Infiltration by lymphocytes, parakeratotic cells, and neutrophils and increase of glycoprotein probably contribute to the formation of the salmon spots.

Onycholysis

This is due to the detachment of the nail plate from the nail bed, due to the inflammation of the latter. Onycholysis initially develops distally or laterally and gradually advances proximally toward the nail

TABLE 2.1

Signs of Psoriasis

Matrix involvement	Nail bed involvement	Fold involvement
Pits, trachyonychia	Onycholysis	Paronychia
Leukonychia	Oil-drop sign	Nail plate disorders
Nail fragility	Splinter hemorrhages	
Dystrophic alterations	Subungual hyperkeratosis	
Beau's lines		
Onychomadesis		
Mottled redness in the lunula		

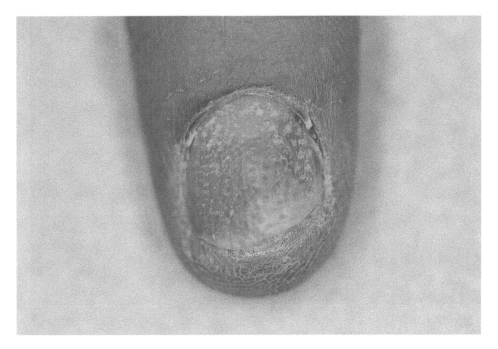

FIGURE 2.1   Pitting on the proximal nail plate associated with distal onycholysis.

matrix. An erythematous border around the onycholytic area in fingernails is diagnostic of psoriasis (Figure 2.4).

Splinter Hemorrhages

Thin longitudinal brown-black lines, about 2–3 mm long, are located distally on the nail plate. They are due to the psoriatic inflammation of the nail bed capillaries and are mainly seen on the fingernails. This is not characteristic of nail psoriasis (Figure 2.5).

Paronychia

Involvement of the paronychial area by psoriatic lesions leads to a secondary phase with complete destruction of the nail plate, due to the inflammation of the underlying matrix (Figure 2.6).

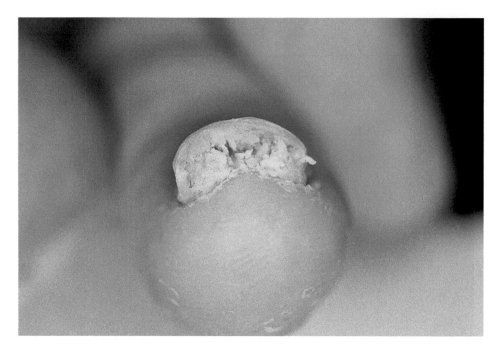

FIGURE 2.2   Subungual hyperkeratosis.

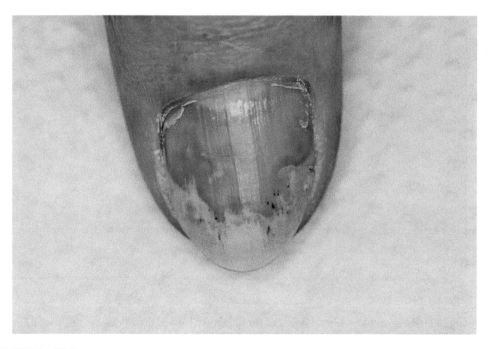

FIGURE 2.3   Oil-drop sign.

Diagnosis

Diagnosis is based on the clinical appearance of the lesions, which are rather characteristic of the disease, especially onycholysis with erythematous border, oil drops, hyperkeratosis, and pits.

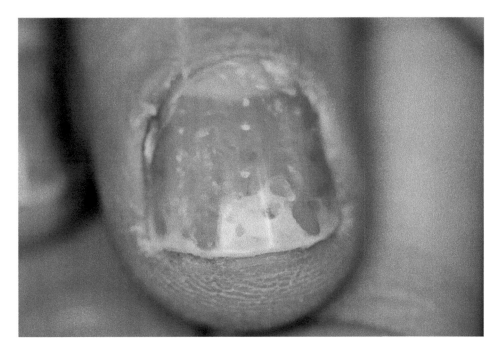

FIGURE 2.4   Onycholysis associated with some pits.

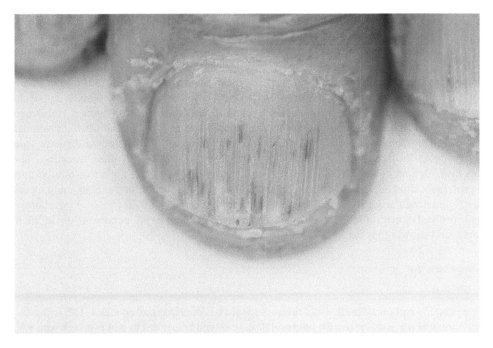

FIGURE 2.5   Splinter hemorrhages.

Existence of psoriasis in other sites of the body can help the clinicians, as can also family or personal history of psoriasis. In doubtful cases, biopsy can prove the diagnosis. However, many clinical features of nail psoriasis are not disease-specific, and several diagnostic tools have been found to be especially helpful to confirm the diagnosis. Several methods and diagnostic techniques

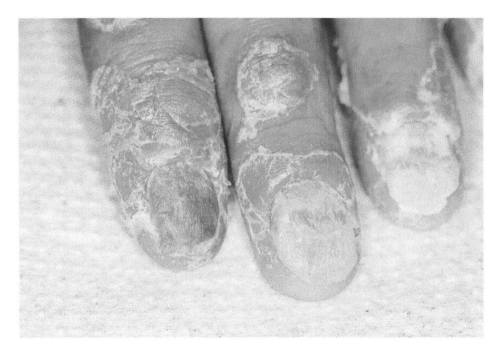

FIGURE 2.6 Paronychia associated with nail dystrophy.

have developed the recent year in order to help confirmation of the disease. Histopathology (it is important to remember that matrix lesions cause changes on the nail plate, while those of the nail bed are seen under the nail plate). Dermoscopy (in cases of onycholysis as the only sign present, dermoscopy can be useful in diagnosis, showing a white homogeneous area. Multiple thin longitudinal white striae might also be visible. It also allows seeing the erythematous border as a red or orange discoloration surrounding the onycholytic areas). Videodermoscopy (capillaries of the hyponychium of nails affected by psoriasis are visible, dilated, tortuous, elongated, and irregularly distributed). Nailfold capillaroscopy (shows the dilated tortuous capillaries of the proximal nail fold). Ultrasonography (may reveal hypervascularity in the nail bed, increased distance from the ventral plate to the bony margin of the distal phalanx, increased nail plate thickness, and enthesopathy). Optical coherence tomography (able to demonstrate even higher resolution changes, with prominent thickening in the ventral plate at the nail bed, which presents as inhomogeneous, "eroded" and irregularly fused). Nail clippings (important differential diagnosis of onychomycosis: in nail psoriasis, neutrophils are mostly aggregated (57.1%) with parakeratosis in increased amounts, and showing no predominant pattern).

Evaluation

When evaluating nail psoriasis, few nail diseases should be defined as nail psoriasis if affecting ≤3 nails. When evaluating fingernail psoriasis, mild nail disease should be defined as nail psoriasis with a NAPSI score of <20.

When evaluating nail psoriasis severity, minimal nail disease should be defined as nail psoriasis with a severity index score of <10% of the maximum used score, mild nail disease should be defined as nail psoriasis with a severity index score of 10%–25% of the maximum used score, moderate nail disease should be defined as nail psoriasis with a severity index score of 26%–50% of the maximum used score, and severe nail disease should be defined as nail psoriasis with a severity index score of >50% of the maximum used score.

Prognosis

Nail psoriasis has an unpredictable course, with remission and relapses, as happens with skin disease. Patients with nail involvement should know that sun exposure often aggravates their disease, as does trauma (the Koebner phenomenon).

Treatment

Simple nail care is important for patients with nail psoriasis.

More treatments (Table 2.2) have been introduced for psoriasis than those for virtually all the rest of dermatology put together. Despite recent therapeutic advances, management of nail psoriasis remains protracted, tedious, and sometimes unsatisfactory. Therefore, treatment of nail psoriasis is a difficult challenge for the clinician to treat.

Treatment for nail psoriasis can be either topical or administered systemically.

The clinician should know that topical treatment for nail psoriasis is not as efficient as in skin disease, because the nail plate prevents drug penetration. Another important point is that it takes a long time (3–9 months) for noticeable nail improvement, due to the slow growth rate of the nail, and the patient should be informed accordingly.

Before the introduction of any treatment, some directions should be given to the patients concerning hand and nail care. Patients should use gloves and even better with cotton ones underneath, especially when they are involved in wet work or come in contact with irritant fluids. They should use nail moisturizers and avoid any trauma, such as over-rigorous manipulations, and they should also keep their nails short, in order to avoid any exacerbation of onycholysis.

They should avoid removing debris from beneath the nail with any instrument. They are allowed to use colored nail enamel, but they should avoid polish removers with formaldehyde-acetone and toluene and, finally, they should avoid artificial nails.

Topical Treatment

Topical treatment is indicated when it is not associated with severe skin psoriasis or psoriatic arthritis, when systemic treatment is not recommended, or in combination with systemic treatment.

TABLE 2.2

Treatment Algorithm

Clinical signs	1st treatment choice	2nd treatment choice
Pits, trachyonychia, proximal leukonychia, lunula with pits	No treatment	Smoothing lacquer (15% urea)
Isolated onycholysis or polydactylous with or without cutaneous involvement	Removal of onycholysis and clobetasol or combination of betamethasone and calcipotriol	Removal of onycholysis and tazarotene
Isolated hyperkeratosis	Injection of triamcinolone (40% urea before)	Calcipotriol
Polydactylous hyperkeratosis	Acitretin 0.5 mg/kg	MTX 15–20 mg/week
Nail ps with joint involvement	MTX 5–10 mg/week	Biologics
Hallopeau	Acitretin 0.3 mg/kg	Retinoid-PUVA

Note: ps, psoriasis.

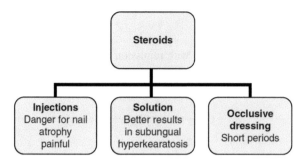

FIGURE 2.7   Treatment with steroids.

- Corticosteroids
- Vitamin D analogs
- Calcipotriol + betamethasone
- Tazarotene
- Tacrolimus
- Fluorouracil 1% solution in propylene glycol and urea (not in use anymore)
- Cyclosporine oily solution (not in use anymore)
- Anthralin (not in use anymore)

Corticosteroids (Figure 2.7)

Potent or superpotent topical steroids can be used once daily (at night) under occlusion. They should be used for 4–6 months and they should be applied to the nail plate, at the hyponychium at the nail folds and at the nail bed, in case the onycholytic nail plate is clipped back. Long-term and repeated use can lead to nail fold atrophy, telangiectasias, and atrophy of the underlying phalanx (disappearing digit). Topical treatment with corticosteroids is unable to act properly in case of subungual hyperkeratosis. Therefore, nail debridement, using 40% urea under occlusion, allows treatment of the nail bed, after removal of the pathological area. Intralesional steroids should follow patients' counseling. Sometimes, topical anesthesia with freezing spray or distal block is needed, and this depends on the patient, the technique, and the size of the needle. A 30-gauge needle locked to the syringe should be used. Triamcinolone acetonide, in a frequency of monthly injections for 5–6 months, is the medication of choice. The injection site depends on the clinical symptom that we are trying to treat (nail matrix or nail bed). Should Dermojet be used for intralesional treatment? Most experts have abandoned this modality due to sterilization problems of the apparatus and also because of the possibility of 'splash back' of small quantities of blood at the time of injecting.

Vitamin D Analogs

Calcipotriol has been used on a twice-a-day basis, for up to 4 to 6 months on the nail plate, hyponychium, nail bed (with the onycholytic nail clipped back), and on the nail folds. According to a paper published by Tosti and others, the use of calcipotriol resulted in 49% reduction of fingernail and 40% of toenail hyperkeratosis.

Calcipotriol, 5 days a week, with clobetasol propionate twice a week, on the nail plate, nail folds, and hyponychium, have been used in a paper published in 2002, with excellent results after 6 and 12 months of patient evaluation (72% improvement in the 6th month, and 81% after 12 months, on the fingernails and 70%, which increased to 73%, on the toenails, over the same period of time).

Tacalcitol and calcitriol have similar efficacy with calcipotriol.

Tacrolimus

Twenty-five patients with nail psoriasis were tried on a combination of calcipotriol and betamethasone ointment every night for 12 weeks. A reduction in the mean Nail Psoriasis Severity Index (NAPSI) score up to 72% was seen at the end of the study period.

Tazarotene

Tazarotene, which is a synthetic retinoid in the form of gel 0.1%, was used in three papers, with very good results. It was used either with or without occlusion, for up to 3 to 8 months. Improvement involved onycholysis, salmon patches, hyperkeratosis, and pitting. In all papers, tolerability was excellent, with only mild skin irritation and a sense of burning or desquamation of the paronychial area. It has been proven superior when compared to clobetasol cream 0.05% under occlusion for 12 weeks.

Tacrolimus

Tacrolimus 0.1% ointment has been proven effective for both nail matrix and bed signs.

Fluorouracil

Since 1998, when the use of 1% 5-FU solution in propylene glycol, with the addition of urea 20%, was reported; there is no other publication and it is not used anymore.

Cyclosporin Solution

Our personal experience is that this medication, despite the good results of one published paper, does not have any effect on nail psoriasis.

Anthralin

Since patients exhibited undesired but reversible, pigmentation of the nail plate; it is no longer used.

Systemic Treatment

Systemic treatment is indicated in the case of the involution of many nails and in the case of pustular psoriasis of the nails (acrodermatitis continua of Hallopeau).

Systemic treatment can be used with the addition of topical treatment in order to reduce the dosage of systemic treatment, or the duration of systemic treatment and also in order to maintain the accomplished remission.

- Retinoids
- Methotrexate
- Cyclosporin
- Biological agents and small molecule drugs
- Laser and light therapies

The clinician should always remember that psoriatic nails can easily be infected by dermatophytes, so the exclusion of this infection, by direct microscopy or culture, must be kept in mind.

Retinoids

Acitretin should be administered at a lower dose than that used in skin psoriasis, 0.3–0.5 mg/kg, in order to avoid the side effects related to retinoids, such as nail fragility, reduction of nail thickness, paronychia-like lesions, and pseudopyogenic granulomas. Etretinate was prescribed in 46 patients with pustular psoriasis with excellent results.

Acitretin was prescribed in 36 patients with nail psoriasis, and it was given at a low dosage, 0.2–0.3 mg/kg, for 6 months. After treatment, the mean percentage reduction of NaPSI was 41%. Clinical evaluation at 6 months showed complete or almost complete clearing of the nail lesions in 25% of the patients, moderate improvement in 25%, mild improvement in 33%, and no improvement in 11% of the patients.

> Systemic treatments have toxicity concerns.

Methotrexate

Methotrexate is recommended to treat nail psoriasis in doses up to 15 mg/week, with proper monitoring until at least moderate improvement has been demonstrated. In cases of coexisting PsA, the methotrexate dosage should be adjusted accordingly. In a study, decrease in NAPSI ranges between 30% and 50% at 52 weeks.

Intralesional MTX has been used, with injections of 2.5 mg/every 30 days for 3 months resulting in significant improvement.

Cyclosporin

Cyclosporin can also improve psoriatic lesions on the nails. In a paper published in 2004, the combination of cyclosporine per os and calcipotriol appeared to be more effective than cyclosporine by itself (47% vs 79% improvement). It has been employed with a dosage of 3 mg/kg followed by either the increase of the dosage to 5 mg/kg/day where needed, or tapering of the dosage during the next 12 weeks.

> - Do not trim nails severely as Koebner's phenomenon can aggravate psoriasis.
> - Onycholysis and pitting are the least responsive to steroid injections.
> - Subungual hyperkeratosis and pitting are responsive to topical fluorouracil, but not onycholysis.
> - 8% clobetasol nail lacquer is effective for onycholysis, pitting, and oil drops.
> - Relapses are common and therapies may need to be maintained or repeated.

Biologics and Small Molecule Drugs

Over the last years, biologics and small molecule drugs have been added to the therapeutic use of dermatologists for psoriasis.

Up to now, there have been a few publications concerning the treatment of nail psoriasis with these medications. However, the major question, concerning the use of these expensive drugs is whether the clinician can use them in psoriasis located only on nails. This question is difficult to answer but in my personal opinion, a useful criterion should be the impact of the nail disease on the quality of life of the patient.

In Table 2.3, the results of different publications are listed.

Apremilast

Apremilast, a selective PDE4 inhibitor, has been proven effective in nail psoriasis. At week 52, a reduction of NAPSI score of 60.2% and 59.7% was observed in ESTEEM 1 and ESTEEM 2 studies.

TABLE 2.3

Efficacy of Biologics on Nails

Etanercept
    57% reduction of NAPSI after 12 months
Adalimumab
    57% reduction of NAPSI after 3 months
    91% reduction of NAPSI after 5 months
Infliximab
    57% reduction of NAPSI at week 14
    94% reduction of NAPSI at week 38
Certolizumab Pegol
    For patients with baseline nail disease (73.3%), mNAPSI change from baseline at week 24 was −1.6 with CZP 200 mg Q2W and −2.0 with CZP 400 mg Q4W versus −1.1 with placebo (p = 0.003 and p < 0.001, respectively)
Golimumab
    43% reduction of NAPSI after 3 months
    54% reduction of NAPSI after 6 months
Guselkumab
    53% reduction of NAPSI after 6 months
Ustekinumab
    50% reduction of NAPSI after 6 months
    90% reduction of NAPSI after 8 months
Secukinumab
    63% reduction of NAPSI at week 32
Ixekizumab
    53% reduction of NAPSI after 5 months

Note: NAPSI, Nail Psoriasis Severity Index.

Similar improvements in NAPSI were observed in the LIBERATE and APPRECIATE studies with 50% of the patients achieving a NAPSI score of 0. Real-world data confirm these results.

Tofacitinib

Tofacitinib is an oral JAK inhibitor. By week 52, 22.2% and 47.6% of the patients who received tofacitinib 5 and 10 mg, respectively, achieved a NAPSI score of 75 in a Japanese randomized, placebo-controlled phase 3 trial.

Etanercept

Etanercept, a fully human TNF-a receptor fusion protein, has been established as a safe and efficacious treatment in nail psoriasis. A dosage of 25 mg twice/week resulted in improvement of NAPSI by 51% at week 24, while a higher dose of 50 mg twice/week for 12 weeks followed by 50 mg once/week for 12 more weeks, showed that NAPSI 75 was reached by 57.0% of the patients.

Adalimumab

The TNF-α inhibitor adalimumab is considered an effective and safe and biologic for treating nail psoriasis, additionally offering rapid results. Patients treated with adalimumab achieved a 57% decrease in the mean NAPSI score at week 12 and a 91% decrease at week 20.

Infliximab

Significant and rapid improvement in nail psoriasis has been revealed with Infliximab, the chimeric monoclonal antibody that also inhibits TNF-α. A decrease in the NAPSI score has been reported to range between 80% and 90% by week 22.

Certolizumab Pegol

In the RAPID study, in patients with psoriatic arthritis treated with certolizumab pegol (a TNF-α inhibitor) was noted a statistically significant improvement of median NAPSI at week 24.

Golimumab

In patients with psoriatic arthritis treatment with golimumab, a human monoclonal antibody against TNF-a, resulted in improvement of median NAPSI by 25% and 33% at weeks 12 and 24 for patients receiving 50 mg of golimumab and 43% and 54% at weeks 12 and 24 for patients receiving 100 mg.

Guselkumab

Two multi-center, randomized, double-blind, placebo, and comparator-controlled clinical trials showed that 27.4% of the patients achieved complete fingernail clearance by week 24 having a similar efficacy to the comparator group receiving adalimumab.

Ustekinumab

Ustekinumab, an IL12/23 inhibitor, has been established as an efficacious and well-tolerated treatment of nail psoriasis. A significant improvement of the NAPSI score is observed by week 12 in patients receiving either 45 mg or 90 mg (depending on body weight) of ustekinumab, highlighting the drug's early efficacy.

Secukinumab

Secukinumab, an IL-17 inhibitor, demonstrated significant and clinically meaningful efficacy and quality-of-life improvements for patients with nail psoriasis up to week 32. The NAPSI percentage change reached −63.2% and −52.6% for secukinumab 300 mg and 150 mg, respectively.

Ixekizumab

Ixekizumab is an IL-17A receptor blocker. In a multiple-dose regimen trial, patients with nail psoriasis in the 75 mg and 150 mg ixekizumab groups had significant improvement from baseline NAPSI. By week 48, 51.0% of patients with nail psoriasis experienced complete resolution of lesions.

Brodalumab

Brodalumab is also an IL-17 receptor blocker with an on-label use in psoriasis. A case series of 4 patients with nail psoriasis reported significant improvement after treatment with brodalumab.

Laser and Light Therapies

In a published study, pulsed dye laser (595 nm), once a month, for 3 months and with a pulse duration of 1.5 ms, beam diameter of 7 mm, and laser energy between 8.0 and 10.0 J/cm appears to be effective particularly in improving onycholysis and subungual hyperkeratosis in a small number of patients.

In another study, with 20 patients, it was found to be an efficacious and well-tolerated option in the treatment of both nail bed and nail matrix psoriasis, after 6 months.

In a pilot study, with 14 patients, the comparison of pulsed dye laser vs photodynamic therapy in the treatment of refractory nail psoriasis has shown that both treatments are equally effective.

Intense pulse light (IPL) treatment was reported, rather promising effective treatment modality, safe and easy to perform.

Excimer laser was compared in a single-blinded left-to-right study versus PDL in patients with nail psoriasis. The results of the excimer laser in nail psoriasis were poor.

Sun can aggravate nail psoriasis.

Phototherapy and Psoralens

PUVA has been reported to improve onycholysis, salmon patches, subungual hyperkeratosis, proximal paronychia, and onychorrhexis in a small series of patients with nail psoriasis. It has no effect on pitting. Given that the nail plate completely blocks UV-B and nearly all UV-A (mean fingernail penetration rate of 1.65%), it is not surprising that UV light treatments for nail psoriasis have been unsuccessful.

Superficial X-Ray Therapy

This treatment modality is still in use in Germany and Switzerland.

FURTHER READING

Abe M., Nishigori C., Torii H., Ihn H., Ito K., Nagaoka M., et al. 2017 Tofacitinib for the treatment of moderate to severe chronic plaque psoriasis in Japanese patients: subgroup analyses from a randomized, placebo-controlled phase 3 trial. *J Dermatol*; 44: 1228–1237.

Aldahan A. S., Chen L. L., Fertig R. M., et al. 2017 Jan Optical coherence tomography for assessment of epithelialization in a human ex vivo wound model. *Skin Appendage Disord*; 2(3–4): 102–108.

Al-Mutairi N., Noor T., Al-Haddad A. 2014 Single blinded left-to-right comparison study of excimer laser versus PDL for the treatment of nail psoriasis. *Dermatol Ther*; 4: 197–205.

Balbas-Marquez M., Sanchez-Regana M., Millet-Umbert P. 2009 Tacalcitol ointment for the treatment of nail psoriasis. *J Dermatol Treat*; 20(5): 308–310.

Baran R. 2004 A nail psoriasis severity index. *Br J Dermatol*; 150: 568–569.

De Berker D. 2000 Management of nail psoriasis. *Clin Exp Dermatol*; 25: 357–362.

De Simone C., Maiorino A., Tassone F., et al. 2013 Tacrolimus 0,1% ointment in nail psoriasis: a randomized, controlled, open-label study. *JEADV*; 27: 1003–1006.

Duarte A. A., Carneiro G. P., Murari C. M., de Jesus L. S. B. 2019 Nail psoriasis treated with intralesional methotrexate injections. *Ann Bras Dermatol*; 94(4): 482–488.

Fernández-Guarino M., Harto A., Sánchez-Ronco M., et al. 2009 Pulsed dye laser vs. photodynamic therapy in the treatment of refractory nail psoriasis: a comparative pilot study. *JEADV*; 23: 891–895.

Golińska J., Sar-Pomian M., Rudnicka L. 2019 (Apr) Dermoscopic features of psoriasis of the skin, scalp and nails – a systematic review. *JEADV*; 33(4): 648–660.

Gumusel M., Ozdemir M., Mevlitoglou I., et al. 2011 Evaluation of the efficacy of methotrexate and cyclosporine therapies on psoriatic nails: a one-blind, randomized study. *JEADV*; 25: 1080–1084.

Iorizzo M., Dahdah M., Vincenzi C., Tosti A. 2008 (Apr) Videodermoscopy of the hyponychium in nail bed psoriasis. *JAAD*; 58(4): 714–715.

Kavanaugh A., McInnes I., Mease P., Krueger G. G., Gladman D., Gomez Reino J. et al. 2009 Golimumab, a new human tumor necrosis factor alpha antibody, administered every 4 weeks as a subcutaneous injection in psoriatic arthritis: 24-week efficacy and safety results of a randomized, placebo-controlled study. *Arthritis Rheum*; 60(4): 976–986.

Kole L., Cantrell W., Elewski B. 2014 Aug A randomized, double-blinded trial evaluating the efficacy and tolerability of vectical ointment (calcitriol 3 mcg/g ointment) when compared to betamethasone diproprionate ointment (64 mg/g) in patients with nail psoriasis *J Drugs Dermatol*; 13(8): 912–915.

Langley G. R., Rich P., Menter A., Krueger G., Goldblum O., Dutronc Y., et al. 2015 Improvement of scalp and nail lesions with ixekizumab in a phase 2 trial in patients with chronic plaque psoriasis. *JEADV*; 29: 1763–1770.

Luger T. A., Barker J., Lambert J., et al. 2009 Sustained improvement in joint pain and nail symptoms with etanercept therapy in patients with moderate-to-severe psoriasis. *JEADV*; 23: 896–904.

Mease P. J., Fleischmann R., Deodhar A. A., Wollenhaupt J., Khraishi M., Kielar D., et al. 2014 Effect of certolizumab pegol on signs and symptoms in patients with psoriatic arthritis: 24-week results of a phase 3 double-blind randomized placebo-controlled study (RAPID-PsA) *Ann Rheum Dis*; 73: 48–55.

Nakamura M., Lee K., Jeon C., Sekhon S., Afifi L., Yan D. 2017 Sep Guselkumab for the Treatment of Psoriasis: A Review of Phase III Trials. *Dermatol Ther (Heidelb)*; 7(3): 281–292.

Neves J. M., Cunha N., João A., Lencastre A. 2019 Nov Neutrophils in nail clipping histology: a retrospective review of 112 cases. *Skin Appendage Disord*; 5(6): 350–354.

Ojeda R., Sanchez-Regana M., Massana J., et al. 2005 Clinical experience with the use of cyclosporine A in psoriasis: results of a retrospective study. *J Dermatol Treat*; 16: 338–341.

Oram Y., Karincaog. lu Y., Koyuncu E., et al. 2010 Pulsed dye laser in the treatment of nail psoriasis. *Dermatol Surg*; 36: 377–381.

Ortonne J. P., Baran R. 2010 Development and validation of nail psoriasis quality of life scale (NPQ10). *JEADV*; 24: 22–27.

Ortonne J. P., Paul C., Berardesca E., Marino V., Gallo G., Brault Y., et al. 2013 A 24-week randomized clinical trial investigating the efficacy and safety of two doses of Etanercept in nail psoriasis. *Br J Dermatol*; 168: 1080–1087.

Parrish C. A., Sobera J. O., Robbins C. M., et al. 2006 Alefacept in the treatment of psoriatic nail disease: a proof of concept study. *J Drugs Dermatol*; 5: 339–340.

Pinter A., Bonnekoh B., Hadshiew I. M., Zimmer S. 2019 Brodalumab for the treatment of moderate-to-severe psoriasis: case series and literature review. *Clin Cosmet Investig Dermatol*; 12: 509–517.

Reich K., Sullivan J., Arenberger P., Mrowietz U., Jazayeri S., Augustin M., et al. 2018 Oct 26. Effect of secukinumab on the clinical activity and disease burden of nail psoriasis: 32-week results from the randomized placebo-controlled TRANSFIGURE trial. *Br J Dermatol* doi: 10.1111/bjd.17351 [epub ahead of print].

Rich P., Scher R. 2003 Nail Psoriasis Severity Index: a useful tool for evaluation of nail psoriasis. *JAAD*; 49: 206–212.

Rigopoulos D., Baran R., Chicheb S., et al. 2019 Jul Recommendations for the definition, evaluation, and treatment of nail psoriasis in adult patients with no or mild skin psoriasis: A dermatologist and nail expert group consensus. *JAAD*; 81(1): 228–240.

Rigopoulos D., Gregoriou S., Katsambas A. 2007 Treatment of psoriatic nails with Tazarotene 0.1% gel vs clobetasol propionate 0.05% cream: a double-blind study. *Acta Derm Venereol*; 87(2): 167–168

Rigopoulos D., Gregoriou S., Lazaridou E., et al. 2010 Treatment of nail psoriasis with adalimumab: an open label unblinded study. *JEADV*; 24: 530–534.

Rigopoulos D., Gregoriou S., Makris M., et al. 2011 Efficacy of Ustekinumab in nail psoriasis and improvement in nail-associated quality of life in a population treated with ustekinumab for cutaneous psoriasis: an open prospective unblinded study. *Dermatology* 223(4): 325–329.

Rigopoulos D., Gregoriou S., Stratigos A., et al. 2008 Evaluation of the efficacy and safety of infliximab on psoriatic nails: an unblinded, nonrandomized, open-label study. *Br J Dermatol*; 159: 453–456.

Tawifik A. A. 2014 Novel treatment of nail psoriasis using the IPL: a 1-year follow-up study. *Dermatol Surg*; 1: 1–6.

Trieewittayapoon C., Sigvahamont P., Chanprapaph K., et al. 2012 The effect of different pulse durations in the treatment of nail psoriasis with 595-nm pulsed dye laser: a randomized, doubleblind, intrapatient left-to-right study. *JAAD*; 66: 807–812.

Van den Bosch F., Manger B., Gouplille P., McHugh N., Rodevand E., Holck P., et al. 2010 Effectiveness of Adalimumab in treating patients with active psoriatic arthritis and predictors of good clinical responses for arthritis, skin and nail lesions. *Ann Rheum Dis*; 69: 394–399.

3

Onychomycosis

Dimitris Rigopoulos
Robert Baran

A revised new classification has been proposed in order to modify the basic model and to include subsequent changes such as the following subtypes of fungal nail plate invasion (Figure 3.1). The purpose of the revised classification is to provide a framework to assist selection of treatment, estimate prognosis, and evaluate new diagnostic methods.

1. Distal and lateral subungual onychomycosis (DLSO)

    This is the most common clinical presentation of onychomycosis. It is often a consequence of tinea pedis and is primarily caused by *T. rubrum*.

    It may be associated with four major clinical features whose contribution may vary with individual cases.

    1.1 Subungual hyperkeratosis (Figure 3.2)

    1.2 Onycholysis (Figure 3.3)

    1.3 Paronychia (Figure 3.4)

    1.4 Chromonychia particularly melanonychia (Figure 3.5)

2. Proximal subungual onychomycosis (PSO)

    This is a rare type of onychomycosis, which may occur equally as often in the toenails as in the fingernails. It is mostly caused by T. rubrum and is most common in patients with acquired immunodeficiency syndrome (AIDS).

    2.1 With paronychia

        2.1.1 So-called Candida paronychia (Figure 3.6). Either as a commensal or from the colonization of a previous paronychia.

        2.1.2 True Candida paronychia (very rare), is usually observed in Chronic mucocutaneous candidosis (CMCC) or HIV-positive subjects.

        2.1.3 Nondermatophyte mold paronychia, sometimes associated with leukonychia (e.g., Fusarium) (Figure 3.7).

        2.1.4 Dermatophyte infection (exceptional).

    2.2 Without paronychia

        We call this type PSO. There are three variants of dermatophytic infection:

        2.1.5 Classical PSO (Figure 3.8)

        2.1.6 Proximal transverse subungual onychomycosis (PTSO) presents as a PSO with atypical patterns: striate leuconychia as isolated or multiple (Figure 3.9). Transverse subungual white strips, separated by areas of nail that are both clinically and histologically normal, affecting the same digit. Proximal to distal longitudinal leukonychia affecting a single digit is exceptional.

        2.1.7 Acute PSO: A rapidly developing form of PSO is recorded in patients with human immunodeficiency virus, who usually have a CD4+ cell count of less than 450 cells/mm^3. This acute type of nail invasion involves several digits simultaneously (Figure 3.10).

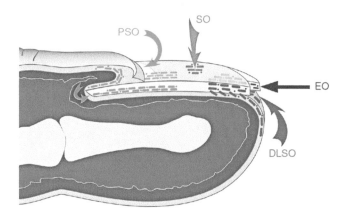

FIGURE 3.1 Different means of nail penetration according to Hay–Baran's revised classification of onychomycosis (2011). Abbreviations: CMC, chronic mucocutaneous candidiasis; DLSO, distal and lateral subungualonychomycosis; EO, endonyxonychomycosis; PWSO, proximal white subungual onychomycosis; PWTSO, proximal white transverse subungual onychomycosis; SWO, superficial white onychomycosis; TDO, total dystrophic onychomycosis.

       2.1.8 Candida PSO has been reported in chronic mucocutaneous candidiasis (CMC).

       2.1.9 Another combination pattern is seen in AIDS patients, where PSO and SO may develop at the same time and spread rapidly to involve the nail plate (see 3.6.2).

3. Superficial onychomycosis (SO)

  This type occurs primarily in the toenails and is usually caused by *T. mentagrophytes* (90% of cases).

  3.1 Classical SO type restricted to the visible NP (Figure 3.11). (There is a black variant)

  3.2 SO from under PNF (Figure 3.12)

  3.3 Acute SO (Figure 3.13)

  3.4 Superficial white transverse onychomycosis (STO) (Figure 3.14)

  3.5 SO with deep invasion (Figure 3.15)

  3.6 Mixed forms with three variants:

      3.6.1 SO associated with DLSO

      3.6.2 SO associated with PSO

      3.6.3 SO associated with histologically restricted involvement of the ventral aspect of the NP (bipolar type)

4. Endonyx onychomycosis (due to *Trichophyton soudanense* but this fungus also causes other forms of onychomycosis) (Figure 3.16).

  The infection penetrates the nail keratin instead of infecting the nail bed. It is most often caused by T. soudanense and T. violaceum, which have high affinity for keratin.

5. Total dystrophic onychomycosis (TDO)

  5.1 Secondary TDO to other forms (Figure 3.17)

    It is the complete progression of any of the above mentioned clinical patterns of onychomycosis.

  5.2 Primary TDO (CMC) (Figure 3.18).

    It only occurs in immunocompromised patients.

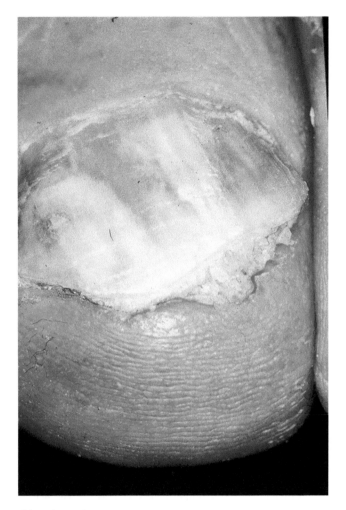

FIGURE 3.2 Subungual hyperkeratosis.

Diagnosis of onychomycosis always requires laboratory confirmation.

Diagnosis

The clinical pattern seen in fungal nail disease only provides a clue to the type of infection. Although certain types of nail involvement are characteristic of certain species, usually the clinical appearance caused by one species of fungus is indistinguishable from that caused by another. Therefore, the diagnosis of onychomycosis always requires laboratory confirmation. However, false-negative mycological results are quite common, especially when samples are taken from a distal nail clipping. Consequently, negative mycology does not completely rule out onychomycosis, since direct microscopy may be negative in up to 20% of cases and cultures may fail to isolate a fungus in up to 30% of cases. Topical antifungals may increase the risk of a false-negative culture. But when the clinical features

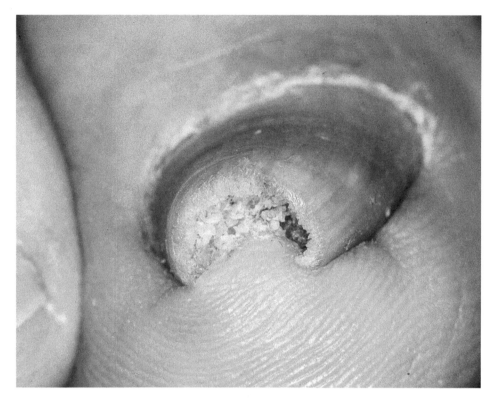

FIGURE 3.3   Onycholysis.

strongly suggest onychomycosis, it is advisable to perform microscopic examination and culture more than once if initial investigations are negative.

In fact, PAS staining is the single method with the highest sensitivity, exceeding that of the gold standard (microscopy and fungal culture) and has been considered as the "new gold standard."

Other techniques that can be used for the diagnosis of onychomycosis are molecular biology (PCR), mass spectrometry (matrix-assisted laser desorption or ionization time-of-flight mass spectrometry MALDI-TOF), flow cytometry, and reflectance confocal microscopy. They require, however, specialized equipment and trained operators, that are generally not easy accessible.

The Dermatophyte Test Strip is a new method, which detects dermatophytes through immunochromatography using monoclonal antibodies that react with polysaccharides present in the cell wall. This antibody was found to react specifically with seven dermatophytes: *T. rubrum*, *T. mentagrophytes*, *T. violaceum*, *T. tonsurans*, *M. gypseum*, *M. canis*, and *E. floccosum*. Further testing should be done to compare this method to microscopy.

How to Collect the Samples

The site of specimen sampling depends on the clinical type of onychomycosis. Separate samples should be obtained from fingernails and toenails. Unfortunately, isolation of a fungus from a nail sample does not necessarily indicate onychomycosis.

The clinician should always bear in mind that some fungi, such as yeasts and most non-dermatophyticmolds, are nail saprophytes rather than pathogens.

Since toenail onychomycosis is frequently associated with tinea pedis, it may be best to collect samples for mycology from the soles. The same rule applies to the palms of patients with fingernail onychomycosis.

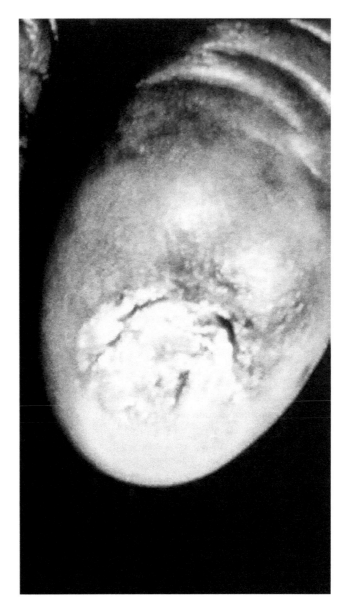

FIGURE 3.4   Paronychia.

Treatment

Systemic Treatment

Griseofulvin is no longer used and Ketoconazole has produced severe cases of hepatotoxicity.

Itraconazole is a triazole that inhibits lanosterol 14α-demethylase in the ergosterol biosynthesis pathway. It is effective on dermatophytes, NDMs, and *Candida* species, and at least *in vitro* has broader spectrum coverage compared to terbinafine. Itraconazole is given as a 200 mg dose once daily for 3 months or as a pulse therapy with intermittent dosing of 200 mg twice daily for 1 week per month over a period of 2 months for fingernails and 3 months for toenails. It is preferably taken with a fatty meal to maximize bioavailability.

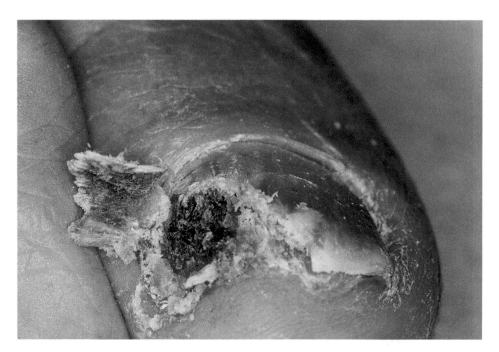

FIGURE 3.5   Fungal melanonychia.

Itraconazole should be avoided during pregnancy and for 2 months before planning pregnancy (Class C) and also during lactation. It is metabolized in the liver by CYP450 3A4 enzyme system and therefore has a long list of potential drug interactions.

Fluconazole, another azole antifungal drug of the triazol group, is mainly used (100 mg daily) in the management of systemic disease and superficial candidiasis, especially in patients with AIDS and in other immunosuppressed subjects as single doses (150 or 300 mg per week for 6–12 months). Fluconazole may provide good control of chronic mucocutaneous candidiasis, particularly in nail involvement. It is approved for the treatment of onychomycosis in Europe and is used commonly off-label in other countries. It is considered a third alternative in dermatophyte onychomycosis, after terbinafine and itraconazole. Its antifungal spectrum covers dermatophytes, *Candida* species, and some NDMs. The recommended dose is 150 mg weekly until the nail has grown out (6–9 months for fingernails, 12–18 months for toenails). Fluconazole can be taken with a meal or on an empty stomach. It should be avoided in pregnant (Class D) and breastfeeding women.

Terbinafine is a member of the allylamine antifungal drug group. Terbinafine is active against a wide range of pathogenic fungi *in vitro*, but *in vivo* is only useful for dermatophytosis 250 mg daily. Significant recovery rates of toenail infections at 3 months and fingernails at 6 weeks. It is considered the gold standard for onychomycosis, with high mycologic (46%–82%) and clinical cure rates (53%–70%) and lower relapse rates compared to other agents. Numerous off-label pulse therapies with terbinafine have been described with efficacy similar to continuous dosing.

Terbinafine can be taken with or without a meal since bioavailability is similar. Use of terbinafine for onychomocosis during pregnancy cannot be recommended (Class B) and due to its excretion into breast milk, it should not be given during the breastfeeding period. It should be noted that it does not inhibit CYP450 3A4, so there is no interaction with the long relevant drug list, including statins.

- Baseline liver function tests are advisable prior to initiating oral antifungal therapy in all patients.
- Immunocompromised patients (e.g., HIV, diabetes, psoriasis) and patients on polypharmacy (e.g., elderly), are more likely to be at risk for drug-to-drug interactions.

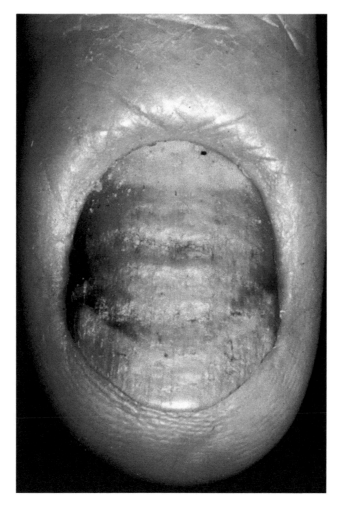

FIGURE 3.6 So-called candida paronychia.

- Terbinafine (continuous) and itraconazole (pulse) are more efficacious than fluconazole. Fluconazole is superior in efficacy to topical treatments.
- A Cochrane review on oral treatments for onychomycosis concluded that terbinafine is likely superior to azoles in terms of efficacy.

Failure Rate

Despite significant improvements with the "new" drugs, at least 20% of patients with onychomycosis still fail on antifungal therapy.

Patients Likely to Fail Therapy

During an adequate nail sampling procedure, where an affected segment of the nail is removed, some clues may anticipate the risk of failure and indicate the best way to eradicate the pathogen: trimming, debridement, nail bed curettage, nail abrasion, and even partial nail avulsion should be considered as an adjunct to antifungal agents.

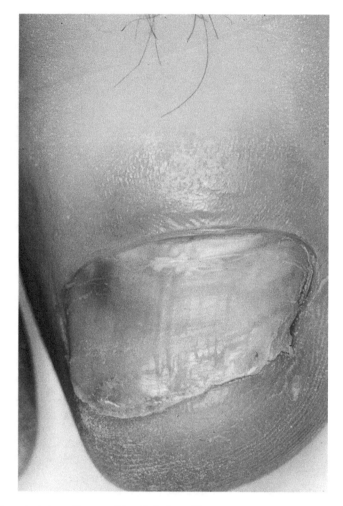

FIGURE 3.7   Nondermatophyte mold paronychia with leukonychia.

Patients with Decrease of Linear Nail Growth

The growth rate in fungally infected nails may be decreased during active infection, especially when more than 50% is involved. The mechanism is not entirely clear, but involvement of both the matrix and nail bed can contribute to slow growth.

Patients with Interruption in the Transport of the Drug

- Onycholysis (extensive)
- Lateral nail disease presenting as lateral onycholysis
- Overthickened nail plate (>2 mm)
- Dermatophytoma as spikes or massive keratin
- Patients with a history of prior infection, men and older patients less likely to reach clinical cure
- Positive culture at 24 weeks affected mycological and clinical cure at 72 weeks negatively

The long-term accumulation of terbinafine and the antifungal azoles enables a relatively short period of treatment for eradication of fungal nail infections. We use (Zaias 1972) terbinafine 250 mg daily 1 week a month for as long as needed.

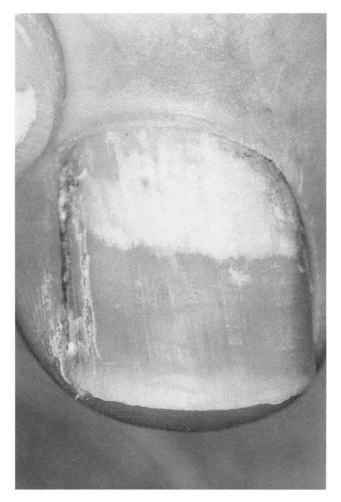

FIGURE 3.8 Classical PSO. (By courtesy of M. Feuilhade.)

Due to the persistence of the drug for 3–6 months after the end of therapy, prolongation of terbinafine treatment duration from 3 to 6 months does not improve mycological and clinical cure rates (Figure 3.19).

Strategies to Improve Efficacy

Supplemental Therapy

There is a window of opportunity for booster therapy until 6–9 months from start of treatment.

Intermittent Treatment

Terbinafine may be an effective treatment for DLSO when 250 mg/day are given 7 days a month for 3 months.

Topical treatment – Transungual Drug Delivery Systems (TUDDS)

Topical monotherapy may be used for onychomycosis affecting less than 50% of the surface area of the nail without matrix involvement and when few nails are affected. The permeability of the drug

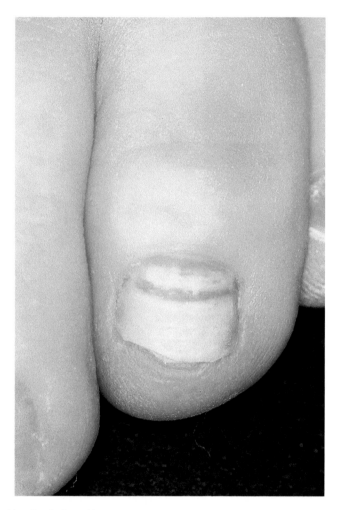

FIGURE 3.9   PSO with striate leukonychia.

through the nail depends on factors such as its molecular weight, lipophilicity, affinity to keratin, ionization, and pH. Topicals are available in two forms: lacquers and solutions. Their transungual penetration and, therefore, efficacy decreases with increasing thickness of the nail. These formulations
fulfill two essential prerequisites. First, the active ingredient is in contact with the nail for long periods.
Second, the concentration of the active ingredient in the remaining film reservoir from which the active
agent is gradually released increases through evaporation of the solvents, thus providing the high
concentration gradient essential for maximal penetration.

Five percent of amorolfine belongs to a new family of antifungal drugs, the morpholines.
Amorolfine inhibits two steps in the pathway of ergosterol biosynthesis, namely the .14-reductase and
the .7,8-isomerase, which play an important role in regulating membrane fluidity. This leads to the
accumulation of abnormal sterols and inhibits fungal growth. Amorolfine possesses a broad anti-
mycotic spectrum against fungi pathogenic to plants and humans. Amorolfine is fungicidal against
yeasts, *Candida albicans*, *Cryptococcus neofromans*, dimorphic and some dematiaceous fungi, but
appears to be less active against Aspergillus, Fusarium, and Mucor. Amorolfine 5% nail lacquer is
applied weekly for 6 months for fingernails and 9 to 12 months for toenails. It is approved in Europe
but not in the United States.

Ciclopirox 8% is a hydroxyl-pyridone derivate with broad-spectrum antimicrobial activity. In contrast
to most antifungals, it does not interfere with sterol biosynthesis. It acts as a chelating agent and

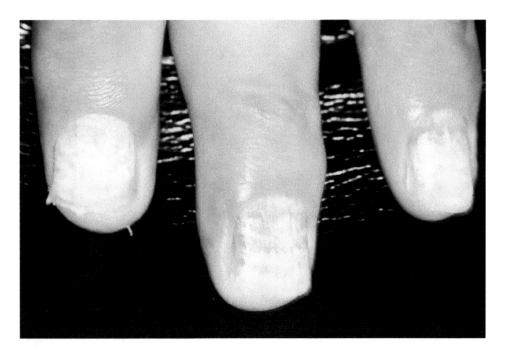

FIGURE 3.10   Acute PSO.

primarily affects iron-dependent mitochondrial enzymes. It inhibits dermatophytes, *Candida* species and some nondermatophyte molds, including *Trichophyton rubrum*, *Epidermophyton* spp., *Candida* spp., and *Scopulariopsis brevicaulis*, as well as a number of Gram-positive and Gram-negative aerobic and anaerobic bacteria. Ciclopirox 8% nail lacquer is FDA approved to treat mild to moderate ony-chomycosis of fingernails and toenails caused by *T. rubrum*. It is applied daily for 24 weeks for fin-gernails and 48 weeks for toenails. The lacquer should be removed weekly with alcohol, and the nails trimmed and filed with an emery board. In addition, monthly clipping by a healthcare professional is recommended to improve efficacy.

Ciclopirox 8% HPCH solution is a hydrolacquer that forms a film over the nail, allowing the solution to penetrate the nail plate. It contains hydroxypropyl chitosan, horsetail extract, and methylsulfonyl methane. This variant of ciclopirox does not necessitate nail abrasion nor does nail enamel remover increase the linear nail growth.

Ciclopirox 8% hydrolacquer is more effective than ciclopirox nail lacquer at week 60 as evaluated in a clinical trial. Ciclopirox hydrolacquer is also more efficacious than amorolfine 5% at week 48 with reported complete cure rates (0% clinical involvement of the nail and negative direct microscopy) of 35% and 11.7%, respectively. It is approved for the treatment of onychomycosis in Europe but not yet in the United States.

Efinaconazole 10% solution was FDA approved as a treatment in 2014. It is a triazole antifungal that inhibits the synthesis of ergosterol in the fungal cell wall. Its indication is the treatment of toenail onychomycosis due to *T. rubrum* and *T. mentagrophytes*. Reported mycological cure rates are 53.4%–55.2% and complete cure rates 15.2%–17.8%. It is applied daily for 48 weeks and no removal, filing, or trimming is necessary.

Tavaborole is a benzoxaborole, and its mechanism of action is inhibition of protein synthesis through fungal aminoacyl transfer RNA synthetase. It exhibits a broad spectrum of activity against dermato-phytes, NDMs, and yeasts. Tavaborole 5% solution was FDA approved in 2014 for the treatment of toenail onychomycosis due to *T. rubrum* and *T. mentagrophytes*. It is applied daily for 48 weeks with no need for removal, trimming, or filing. Mycological cure rates were 31.1% and 35.9% and complete cure rates were 6.5% and 9.1%, respectively.

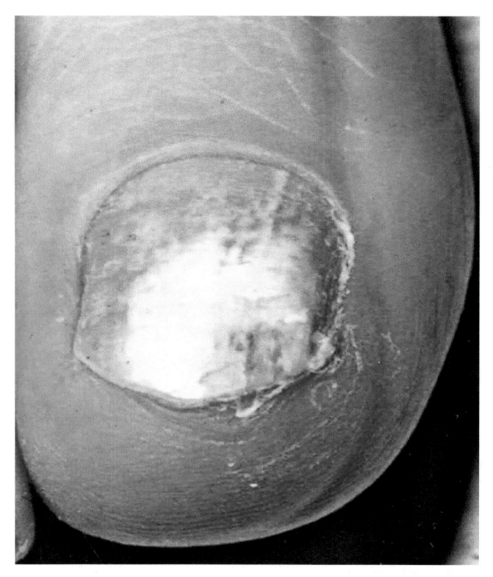

FIGURE 3.11   Classical SO.

Penetration of the drug tioconazole through the plate is excellent but is not matched by clinical efficacy.

All the above topical agents against onychomycosis should not be used during pregnancy or lactation because of unknown safety status.

Advantages of topical treatment:

- No systemic side effects
- No drug-drug interactions
- No need for laboratory monitoring

However, efficacy remains low.

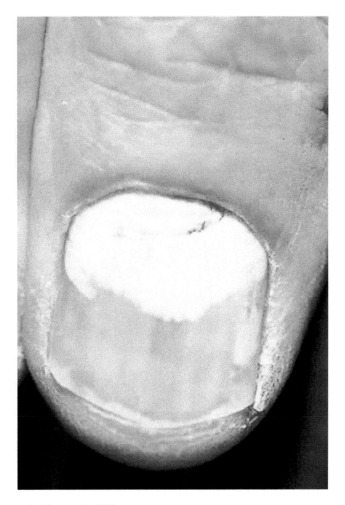

FIGURE 3.12 SO emerging from under PNF.

Mechanical Interventions and Role of Nail Surgery in the Treatment of Onychomycosis

Surgery can be useful in the treatment of onychomycosis. Nail avulsion is helpful particularly under occlusion, but only as an adjunct to oral and/or topical antifungal agent. It is the logical way to best eradicate the pathogen, especially in patients likely to fail. For example, in dermatophytoma, the sequestered area of nail keratin does not permit penetration of the drug. In addition to dermatophyte nail infection, nail plate avulsion is very helpful in treating onychomycosis caused by molds.

Total surgical removal has to be discouraged: the distal nail bed may shrink and become dislocated dorsally. In addition, the loss of counterpressure produced by the removal of the nail plate allows expansion of the distal soft tissue, and the distal edge of the regrowing nail then embeds itself. This can be largely overcome by using partial nail avulsion, which can be performed under local anesthesia, in a selected group of patients in whom the fungal infection is limited. It permits the removal of the affected portion of the nail plate in one session, even when the disease has reached the buried region of the subungual tissue, beneath the proximal nail fold. Total surgical removal is contraindicated for patients with diabetes mellitus, vascular diseases, autoimmune diseases, and disorders of hemostasis.

In DLSO, partial surgical removal consists of sectioning the lateral or medial segment of the nail plate. Therefore, enough normal nail is left to counteract the upward forces exerted on the distal soft tissue when walking, and this will prevent the appearance of a distal nail wall.

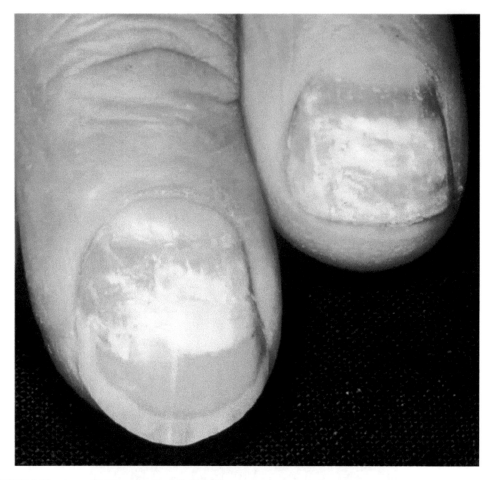

FIGURE 3.13   Acute SO. (By courtesy of C. Gianni.)

In Candida onycholysis, a thorough clipping away of as much of the detached nail as possible facilitates the daily application of antifungal drug until nail growth is achieved. In PSO, removal of the nonadherent base of the nail plate cut transversely leaves the distal portion of the nail in place, which decreases discomfort. Recalcitrant Candida paronychia with secondary nail plate invasion may be treated by surgical excision of a crescent of thickened nail fold. In any type of onychomycosis treated surgically, the avulsed segment must always include a margin of normal nail.

Good results have been obtained recently by combining surgical techniques with either intermittent or short duration use of new oral antifungal drugs.

In patients at risk (immunosuppressive conditions, immunosuppressive therapy, peripheral vascular disease), chemical avulsion is a painless method that has superseded partial surgical avulsion. It may be repeated as often as necessary. Forty percent urea ointment appears to focus its action on the bond between the nail keratin and the diseased nail bed; it spares the normal nail tissue.

Management of Various Subtypes

In primary onycholysis of big toenails, associated with dermatophyte invasion, measures should be taken to relieve the effects of pressure and trauma, such as the provision of fitted shoes, padding, and toe shields. Topical treatment with antifungal therapy and repeated trimming of the nonadherent portion of the nails should be started.

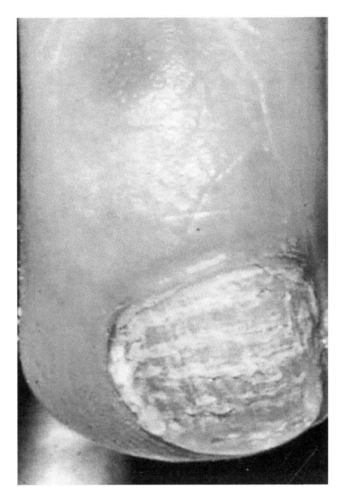

FIGURE 3.14 Superficial white transverse onychomycosis.

Superficial white onychomycosis caused by dermatophytes should be abraded (sandpapered) after confirming the diagnosis. When the culture is negative, the shaving technique of the dorsum of the nail or a 3-mm punch biopsy restricted to the plate is taken for histopathology. When superficial white onychomycosis (SWO) emerges from beneath the cuticle, combination therapy is mandatory.

Nondermatophyte Mold Onychomycosis

Assuming that the pathogenic role of mold fungi isolated from the affected nails has been confirmed, three patterns of infection should be considered.

1. SWO caused by *Acremonium*, *Aspergillus*, or *Fusarium* spp. involving the visible portion of the nail plate or emerging from beneath the proximal nail fold.
2. DLSO caused by *Scopulariopsis brevicaulis*, *Pyrenochaeta unguium-hominis*, *Scytalidium dimidiatum* and *hyalinum*.
3. Proximal subungual onychomycosis due to *Fusarium* spp.

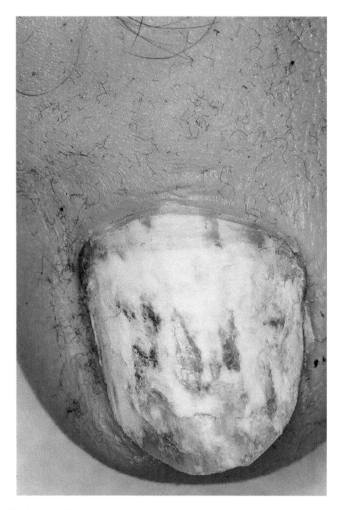

FIGURE 3.15   SO with deep invasion.

Mechanical therapy is indispensable as partial or even total nail avulsion. Any of the three main systemic antifungals may be tried in combination with Whitfield ointment and then followed by nail lacquer applications.

However, good response on *Aspergillus* spp. has been observed with terbinafine 500 mg daily one week monthly for 3 months.

Cases due to *Fusarium* sp., *Acremonium* sp., and *Aspergillus* sp., are often insensitive to standard medications. In these cases, a study by Lurati M and others showed very good results with a solution of amphotericine (DMSO and isopropyl alcohol 1:1) at a final concentration of 2 mg/ml, applied once a day (clinical cure in 8/8 cases, after 12 months of treatment, mycological cure in 7/8 patients). In some cases, urea-based cream was used to enhance penetration of amphotericin solution (must be stored in an amber glass bottle).

Candida Onychomycosis

Candida onychomycosis can be treated with oral itraconazole, fluconazole, topical eficonazole, or chemical removal, with urea followed by local antifungal treatment. If these methods are unsuccessful, partial or complete avulsion and chemotherapy should also be used.

In CMCC, itraconazole and fluconazole are effective.

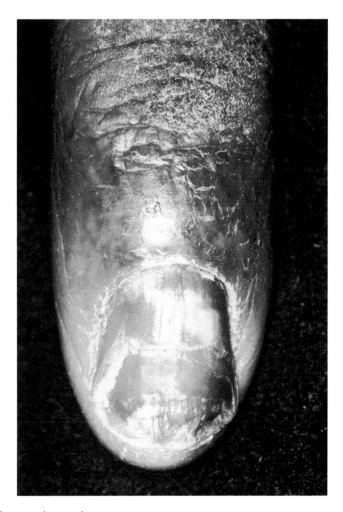

FIGURE 3.16　Endonyxonychomycosis.

Ingrowing Toenails as an Adverse Consequence of Effective Treatment of Onychomycosis

Clinicians should be aware that onychocryptosis may be a potential complication of effective oral treatment for onychomycosis, and the reasons for this is that clinically the therapeutic response is a proximal clearing of the nail plate with resolution of the distal subungual debris. As the healthy nail plate advances, it may adhere to the nail bed, cutting into the lateral nail folds. This could explain the emergence of onychocryptosis.

Sculptured artificial nails or gels are applied on the remaining portion of the plate. When avulsion is total, the preformed artificial plastic nail is applied on the whole nail bed and fixed onto it with a micropore as long as needed. Both types of false nails prevent the heaping up of the distal tissue.

Finally, long-term intermittent therapy might prevent the re-establishment of tinea pedis and limit the risk of nail reinfection. Periodic use of transungual antifungal drug delivery systems, which are retained in nail keratin after discontinuation of therapy, appears to be a logical and safe method for

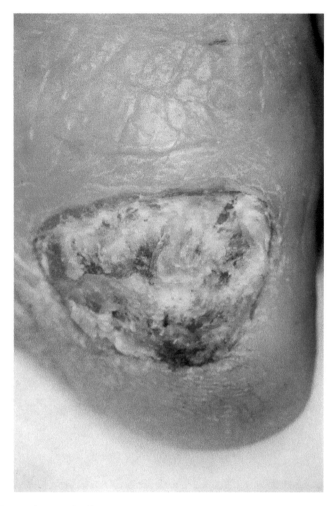

FIGURE 3.17   TDO secondary to other forms.

- Keep nails clean and short.
- Avoid going barefoot in public places.
- Use an antifungal foot powder daily.
- Wear only your own shoes.
- Old, worn footwear should be discarded.
- Wear comfortable, wide, properly fitting shoes.
- Wear cotton rather than synthetic socks.
- Check family members for fungal infections and treat as necessary.
- Prevent tinea pedis.
- Treat/control comorbidities, such as diabetes, vascular disease, neuropathy, obesity.

Confirmation in the efficacy of amorolfine nail lacquer twice a month for the prophylaxis of onychomycosis over 3 years has been published.

Interestingly, ciclopirox water-soluble nail lacquer shows a residue ciclopirox amount of 8.8 μg/mg in the nails, which is three orders of magnitude larger than the MICs for dermatophytes and yeasts.

This allows one to conclude that the active ingredient remains in the nails for at least 4 weeks.

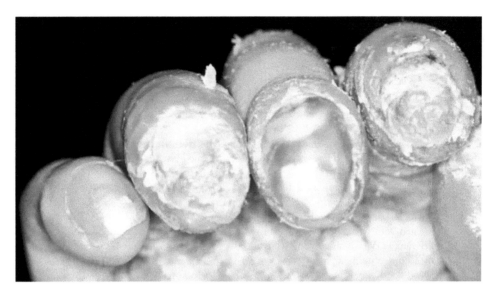

FIGURE 3.18   Primary TDO (CMC).

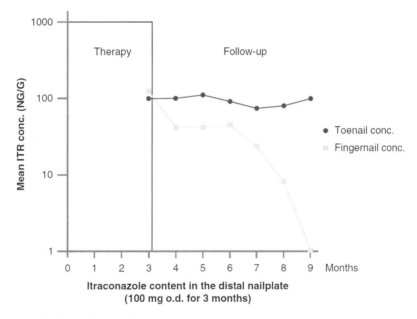

FIGURE 3.19   Terbinafine or itraconazole content.

Combination Therapy

Many studies have demonstrated superiority of combination treatment for onychomycosis. Combining systemic therapy with topicals may achieve a broader antifungal spectrum, possibly synergism, especially with drugs with different mechanism of action. Studies where amorolfine has been paired with itraconazole or fluconazole and terbinafine with ciclopirox confirmed the value of these combinations in moderate to severe cases with negative prognostic factors or with a mixed infection. Nail drilling prior to topical therapy and fractional carbon dioxide laser-assisted therapy are examples of combinations that have improved cure rates. Further clinical studies that systematically investigate the efficacy of combination treatments are recommended.

FURTHER READING

Aditya K. Gupta, Rachel R. Mays, Sarah G. Versteeg, Neil H. Shear, Vincent Piguet (2018): Update on current approaches to diagnosis and treatment of onychomycosis, *Expert Review of Anti-infective Therapy*, DOI: 10.1080/14787210.2018.1544891

Baran R, Hay R, Haneke H, Tosti A. *Onychomycosis*. 2nd edn. Boca Raton. 2006.

Dominguez-Cherit J, Teixeira F, Arenas R. Combined surgical and systemic treatment of onychomycosis. *Br J Dermatol* 1999; 140:778–780.

Epstein E. How often does oral treatment of toenail onychomycosis produce a disease-free nail? An analysis of published data. *Arch Dermatol.* 1998; 134:1551–1554.

Gianni C, Romano C. Clinical and histological aspects of toenail onychomycosis caused by *Aspergillus* spp: 34 cases treated with weekly intermittent terbinafine. *Dermatology* 2004; 209:104–110.

Goodfield MJD, Evans EGV. Combined treatment with surgery and short duration oral antifungal therapy in patients with limited dermatophyte toenail infection. *J Dermatol Treat* 2000; 11:259–262.

Gupta AK, Baran R, Summerbell R. Onychomycosis: strategies to improve efficacy and reduce recurrence. *J EuropAcadDermatolVenereol* 2002; 16:579–586.

Gupta AK, Fleckman P, Baran R. Ciclopirox nail lacquer topical solution 8% in the treatment of toenail onychomycosis. *J Am AcadDermatol* 2000; 43:S70–S80.

Hay R, Baran R. Onychomycosis: a proposed revision of the clinical classification. *J Am AcadDermatol* 2011; 65:1219–1227.

Lurati M, Baudraz-Rosselet F, Vernez M, et al. Efficacious treatment of non-dermatophyte mould onychomycosis with topical amphotericin B. *Dermatology.* 2011; 223(4):289–292.

Marty JP. Amorolfine nail lacquer: a novel formulation. *J EurAcadDermatolVenereol* 1995; 4(Suppl): S17–S22.

Scher RK. Prevention, relapse and cure. *Topical News Onychomycosis* 2001; 3: 1–3.

Shari R. Lipner (2019): Pharmacotherapy for onychomycosis: new and emerging treatments, *Expert Opinion on Pharmacotherapy*, DOI: 10.1080/14656566.2019.1571039

Sigurgeirsson B, Olafsson JH, Steinsson JT, et al. Efficacy of amorolfi ne nail lacquer for the prophylaxis of onychomycosis over 3 years. *JEADV* 2009. [Epub ahead of print].

Sigurgeirsson B, Paul C, Curran D, Evans EVG. Prognostic factors of mycological cure following treatment of onychomycosis with oral antifungal agents. *Br J Dermatol* 2002; 147:1241–1243.

Zaias N. Onychomycosis. *Arch Dermatol* 1972; 105:263–274.

4

Novel and emerging pharmacotherapy and device-based treatments for onychomycosis

Jose W. Ricardo
Shari R. Lipner

Introduction

Treatment of onychomycosis is often challenging for a number of reasons. Given its chemical composition, the nail plate functions as a formidable physical barrier, and achieving adequate penetration to the subungual space, the active site of infection, is difficult. Several months of treatment are usually required to eradicate pathogens, which may limit patient compliance. Furthermore, because fingernails and, particularly, toenails grow exceedingly slowly, visible improvement takes many months, further limiting adherence to therapy. In addition, with oral treatments, there are risks of systemic toxicity, and a number of potential drug-drug interactions. Many patients with onychomycosis have predisposing conditions, such as diabetes, peripheral vascular disease, or immunosuppression that require polypharmacy, therefore limiting effective options for onychomycosis treatment.

Pharmacotherapy

Topical Terbinafine Reformulations

Terbinafine, a synthetic antifungal of the allylamine class, noncompetitively inhibits squalene epoxidase, leading to ergosterol-depleted fungal cell membranes and the toxic accumulation of intracellular squalene. Oral terbinafine is approved by the United States Food and Drug Administration (FDA) for onychomycosis treatment and is considered the gold standard for its excellent efficacy with low incidence of adverse side effects. However, with oral administration, there are risks of systemic toxicity and drug-drug interactions. Theoretically, with sufficient transungual penetration, topical terbinafine may offer similar efficacy without systemic drug uptake, mitigating potential drug interactions and adverse effects.

Terbinafine nail solution (TNS) has undergone three phase III clinical trials to assess its efficacy vs. vehicle and amorolfine 5% nail lacquer for treatment of onychomycosis. Overall, complete cure was not different between TNS and vehicle, and mycological cure was similar in the TNS vs. amorolfine groups. Since terbinafine hydrochloride has poor nail plate penetration, liposomal formulations were examined for their ability to enhance permeation. In comparison with all the tested formulations, with once daily application in rabbit nails, liposome-loaded pullulan LI-P was most effective as its thinner film, remained on the nail plate for 24 hours due to bioadhesive properties, allowing for continuous drug release.

Terbinafine 10% nail solution (MOB-015) was studied in a 52-week multi-center, double-blind, vehicle-controlled phase III study ($n = 365$) to assess efficacy and safety of once-daily application of MOB-015 for 48 weeks vs. vehicle for the treatment of distal and lateral subungual onychomycosis. MOB-015 was significantly more effective in treating dermatophyte toenail onychomycosis compared to vehicle, with a mycological cure (negative direct KOH microscopy and fungal culture of dermatophytes) rate of 69.9%. However, complete cure rate (mycological cure and 0% clinical involvement) was 4.5%, possibly because the vehicle (urea, lactic acid, propylene glycol) resulted in nail discoloration. In comparison, the mycological cure rate for oral terbinafine is 70%, with a complete cure rate of 38%. Adverse events were limited to application site reactions and included blister (0.8%), dermatitis (1.2%), contact dermatitis (2.8%), erythema (0.4%), nail bed bleeding (0.8%), and onycholysis (0.8%); nonetheless, use of MOB-015 was not associated with systemic adverse reactions or drug-drug interactions that are associated with the oral formulation.

TDT-067 is terbinafine enclosed in a Transfersome® particle, which is a lipid aggregate with a hydrophilic exterior designed to increase drug transport across the nail plate. TDT-067 is more effective than conventional terbinafine preparations (oral/topical spray) against *T. mentagrophytes, E. floccosum, T. rubrum,* and terbinafine-resistant *T. rubrum.* It is administered twice daily for 12 weeks. In phase II studies, 1.5% TDT-067 applied twice daily for 12 weeks resulted in a mycological cure rate of 38.5% at week 48.

NB-002 is terbinafine in an oil-in-water emulsion with nanometer-sized droplets. It has better antifungal activity against common dermatophytes involved in onychomycosis as well as *C. albicans.* In a phase II study of patients with mild onychomycosis (≤50% of nail involvement), a 42-week course of NB-002 resulted in a mycological cure in 25%–31.7% of participants at 4 or 8 weeks across three active treatment groups ($n = 227$) (0.25% solution twice daily, 0.5% solution once or twice daily), and treatment was well-tolerated. The rate of effective treatment (mycological cure and ≤10 mm nail involvement or ≥5 mm new growth) ranged from 4.2% to 16.9%.

P-3058 is another innovative terbinafine transungual solution. It is based on a film-forming hydroxypropyl Chitosan technology, which enhances penetration through the nail plate. In a dose investigation study of patients with mild-to-moderate onychomycosis due to dermatophytes, P-3058 5%, o.d., 10% o.d. and 10% o.w. had superior efficacy compared to P-3058 2% after 24 weeks. A multicenter, randomized, double-blind, parallel, vehicle-controlled study assessing efficacy, and safety of P-3058 10% nail solution is being conducted.

The different topical formulations of terbinafine and their main properties are summarized in Table 4.1.

TABLE 4.1

Topical Formulations of Terbinafine and Their Properties

Formulation	Properties/characteristics
Terbinafine nail solution with liposome-loaded pullulan LI-P	Liposomes improve penetration through the nail and allow for continuous drug release. Pullulan, a linear homopolysaccharide of glucose, has bioadhesive properties, which promotes sustained release (24 hours)
Terbinafine 10% nail solution (MOB-015)	Vehicle: urea, lactic acid, propylene glycol. Phase III study ($n = 365$): Mycologic cure: 69.9% Complete cure: 4.5%
TDT-067	Terbinfaine enclosed in a Transfersome particle, a lipid aggregate with a hydrophilic exterior designed to enhance permeability across the nail plate
NB-002	Terbinafine in an oil-in-water emulsion with nanometer-sized droplets. Phase II study ($n = 227$) Mycologic cure: 25–31.7%
P-3058	Terbinafine in hydroxypropyl chitosan, a film-forming agent that enhances penetration through the nail

Newer more effective topical antifungals would theoretically negate the need for systemic treatment, thus reducing potential risks of toxicity and drug-drug interactions.

Azoles

Azole antifungals are the largest class of drugs used in the systemic treatment of onychomycosis. Azole drugs show a moderate level of efficacy in the treatment of onychomycosis, but they are associated with adverse events and drug interactions due to their interactions with cytochrome P450 enzymes. The investigations into new azole molecules with higher efficacy and fewer adverse events have resulted in a number of new molecular entities intended for systemic and topical administration.

Topical Azoles

Bifonazole is a topical triazole molecule that is currently available as a 1% cream formulation in Europe for the topical treatment of onychomycosis. Treatment regimens often include non-surgical nail ablation as an adjunct with urea 40% applied for 2 to 4 weeks before application of bifonazole 1% cream, or urea in combination with bifonazole 1% cream. It has seen renewed interest in North America due to its fungistatic efficacy against *T. rubrum.*

Efinaconazole is a topical triazole antifungal that inhibits lanosterol 14α-demethylase, impeding ergosterol synthesis, and is effective against dermatophytes and yeasts. Its low affinity for keratin and low surface tension allow for favorable penetration through the nail plate. A 10% solution was approved by the US FDA in 2014. Two 52-week prospective, multicenter, randomized, double-blind studies of patients aged ≥18 years assessed efficacy and safety of efinaconazole 10% solution for toenail onychomycosis. Complete cure was achieved in 17.8% of efinaconazole-treated subjects versus 3.3% for vehicle, and 15.2% versus 5.5% ($P < 0.001$) in studies 1 and 2, respectively. In study 1, 55.2% of patients treated with efinaconazole versus 16.8% with vehicle achieved mycological cure, and 53.4% of efinaconazole-treated patients versus 16.9% in the placebo group achieved mycological cure in study 2. Efinaconazole 10% solution has been associated with ingrown nail (2.3%), application site dermatitis (2.2%), vesicles (1.6%), and pain (1.1%). It penetrates human cadaveric nails coated with nail polish.

Luliconazole is an imidazole antifungal that decreases ergosterol synthesis by inhibiting lanosterol demethylase. It has activity against dermatophytes and nondermatophyte molds (NDMs). A cream formulation was approved by the USA FDA since 2013, and in Japan since 2005 for the treatment of superficial mycoses, including tinea pedis; it is not approved for the treatment of onychomycosis. *In vitro,* it was shown to have higher potency than amorolfine, ciclopirox, and topical terbinafine against dermatophytes. It has a high molecular weight, which hinders penetrance through the nail plate; however, a modified molecular structure with reduced keratin affinity allows the drug to be readily released from the nail plate's keratin matrix, thereby enhancing nail permeability. A randomized vehicle-controlled phase III study of onychomycosis patients aged 21–79 years with 20–50% nail involvement was conducted to assess efficacy of luliconazole 5% nail solution. After 48 weeks, 14.9% of patients treated with luliconazole 5% solution applied once daily achieved complete cure compared with vehicle (5.1%, $P = 0.012$). Luliconazole-treated patients also showed significantly higher rates of mycological cure compared with vehicle (45.4% versus 31.2%, $P = 0.026$). Adverse reactions associated with luliconazole were mostly localized, and mild or moderate, including dry skin (6.7%), contact dermatitis (5.2%), paronychia (4.1%) and eczema (3.1%). Therefore, once-daily application of luliconazole 5% solution is clinically effective and well tolerated.

Ketoconazole nanoemulgel containing permeation enhancer was formulated as a vehicle for transungual drug delivery, and its efficacy was investigated *in vitro*. It showed enhanced *in vitro* antifungal activity in *T. rubrum* and *C. albicans* compared to vehicle alone. Since skin irritation and histopathologic studies failed to show clinical and microscopic evidence of skin irritation, it may be a promising formulation for the topical treatment of onychomycosis.

Ketoconazole-encapsulated cross-linked fluorescent supramolecular nanoparticles (KTZ⊂c-FSMNPs) is an intradermal controlled released solution that is a potential treatment for onychomycosis. A variety of KTZ⊂c-FSMNPs was produced using a two-step synthetic approach, and characterization revealed that 4800 nm KTZ⊂c-FSMNPs exhibited high ketoconazole encapsulation efficiency/capacity, optimal fluorescent property, and sustained ketoconazole release profile. *In vivo*, 4800 nm KTZ⊂c-FSMNPs were deposited intradermally *via* tattoo using a mouse model; results demonstrated that 4800 nm KTZ⊂c-FSMNPs functions as an intradermal controlled solution and thus it can potentially serve as an effective treatment for onychomycosis.

Benzoxaboroles

Benzoxaboroles are a new class of antifungal agents based on boron-containing molecules. They inhibit protein synthesis by inhibiting the LeuRS tRNA synthetase. This mechanism of action is unique as most antifungals target cell wall synthesis pathways.

Tavaborole is an oxaborole antifungal, and it inhibits fungal protein synthesis by inhibition of an aminoacyl-transfer ribonucleic acid (tRNA) synthesis (AARS). It is effective against most strains of *T. rubrum* and *T. mentagrophytes*, and a 5% solution was FDA-approved for toenail onychomycosis caused by these microorganisms since July 2014. It also has broad-spectrum antifungal activity against less common dermatophytes, NDMs, and yeasts. Because it has a low molecular weight, it sufficiently penetrates the nail plate; furthermore, it has increased affinity for fungal proteins, limiting interference with host proteins. In two 52-week phase III randomized, double-blind, vehicle-controlled studies, mycological cure was achieved in 31.1% and 35.9% of tavaborole-treated participants in studies 1 and 2, respectively, which was significantly higher than vehicle (7.2% and 12.2%, $P<0.001$). Both studies also showed significantly higher rates of complete cure compared to vehicle (6.5% vs 0.5%, $P=0.001$ for study 1; 9.1% vs 1.5%, $P=0.001$ for study 2). Side effects include application site exfoliation (2.7%), ingrown toenail (2.5%), application site erythema (1.6%), and dermatitis (1.3%).

AN-2718 is another antifungal benzoxaborole molecule with high nail penetration. It has a broad-spectrum antifungal activity against yeasts, dermatophytes, and NDMs. *In vitro*, it has shown comparable efficacy to terbinafine and fluconazole for *T. rubrum, T. mentagrophytes, E. floccosum, M. canis, Candida* spp., and other NDMs.

Other Topical Antifungals

AR-12 (OSU-03012) is a novel celecoxib derivative that has broad-spectrum antifungal activity against dermatophytes, such as *T. rubrum*, and yeasts, including *C. neoformans* and *C. albicans*, and NDMs. Its mechanism of action is not precisely known, but it is thought to inhibit the activity of acetyl CoA synthase in the fungal wall and also downregulates host chaperone proteins, such as 78 kDa glucose-regulated protein (GRP78), HSP90 and HSP27, reducing the host immune response, which in turn, may provide a high genetic barrier to the development of pathogen resistance. In *in vitro* studies using cadaveric human nail plates, dexpanthenol and PEG 400 delivered significant quantities of AR-12 into and across the nail plate that was more than MIC 50 level of the drug.

Auriclosene (NVC-422) is a stable analog of *N*-chlorotaurine, a mild oxidant produced by granulocytes and macrophages during the oxidative burst. NVC-422 has broad-spectrum anti-bacterial and antifungal activity *in vitro*. Using a cadaveric model, NVC-422 in nanoemulsion lacquers and gel formulations showed significant drug penetration and efficacy in inhibiting dermatophyte growth.

ME-1111 is a novel antifungal with potent *in vitro* antifungal activity against dermatophytes, namely *T. rubrum* and *T. mentagrophytes*. It has a low molecular weight, allowing for high permeability through the nail plate, and also has low affinity to keratin. Its antifungal activity is mediated by the inhibition of succinate dehydrogenase (complex II), an important enzyme in the mitochondrial respiratory electron transport chain. Its *in vitro* efficacy as measured in deep nail layers, was significantly higher than that of efinaconazole, tavaborole, ciclopirox, and amorolfine in a phase II randomized, double-blind, vehicle-controlled, dose-ranging study in patients with toenail onychomycosis. *In vitro* and *in vivo* correlation and well-controlled clinical data are needed to confirm these results.

Key characteristics of the main topical antifungal agents are summarized in Table 4.2.

Systemic Azoles

Albaconazole is an investigational triazole that is effective against a broad spectrum of dermatophyte and yeast species. It has a long half-life, which allows for once weekly dosage. In a phase II study, 54% of the patients treated with albaconazole once weekly for 36 weeks had a mycologic cure at week 52 with a favorable safety profile. Therefore, it may be an alternative to existing systemic therapies for distal subungual onychomycosis in the future.

Posaconazole has completed a phase II multicenter, double blind clinical trial for the treatment of onychomycosis. The endpoints were negative culture and complete cure. Posaconazole administered at 400 mg/day or 200 mg/day for 24 weeks had a comparable efficacy to terbinafine administered at 250 mg/day for 12 weeks. The percentage of participants who achieved a mycological cure was 78.8% for 400 mg/day posaconazole, 70.3% for 200 mg/day posaconazole, and 71.4% for 250 mg/day terbinafine. The complete cure rate was 45.5%, 54.1%, and 37% for those three treatment arms, respectively. The most common adverse events reported were diarrhea, nausea, and fatigue. However, the availability of low-cost generic terbinafine may limit posaconazole use to second-line treatment in terbinafine-refractory infections, those with NDM infections or those with contraindications to terbinafine.

Pramiconazole is a novel triazole drug with activity against dermatophytes, *Candida* and *Malassezia in vitro*. Both oral and topical preparations have shown superior efficacy compared to itraconazole and terbinafine against *Microsporum canis* in guinea pigs.

Ravuconazole is a triazole antifungal drug and **fosravuconazole** is one of its prodrugs that has undergone Phase III clinical trials. The most effective dose regimen for fosravuconazole was 100 mg/day, which resulted in 82% mycological cure rates at week 48.

VT-1161 is a novel tetrazole CYP51 inhibitor designed to selectively target fungal enzymes and maintains high potency for the fungal target with low levels of interaction with human CYPs. This may translate to a more favorable side effect profile compared to other azoles. *In vitro* and *in vivo* studies have demonstrated broad-spectrum activity against both Candida species and dermatophytes. In a randomized, phase 2b study, with a daily dosing regimen of 300 mg or 600 mg for 14 days, followed by a once-weekly dose (same strength) for either 10 weeks or 22 weeks, mycological cure was achieved for 61% to 72% of patients at week 48, whereas complete cure rates ranged from 32% to 42%.

Voriconazole is a triazole antifungal that has been approved for the treatment of systemic fungal infections, including candidemia, aspergillosis, and serious infections caused by Fusarium species. It has a broad-spectrum antifungal activity *in vitro*, but it has not been assayed for the treatment of onychomycosis in large scale trials. In a recently published report, a recalcitrant (itraconazole/terbinafine) case of fingernail onychomycosis showed complete response to oral voriconazole after 3 months of treatment.

Novel topical antifungal formulations are being studied for improved efficacy and nail plate penetrability compared to currently available options.

TABLE 4.2

Topical Antifungal Agents

Class	Drug	Formulation	Regimen	Mechanism of action	Molecular weight (g/mol)	Reported cure rate (%)
Allylamine	Terbinafine	MOB-015 (terbinafine 10% nail solution)	Once-daily for 48 weeks	Inhibits squalene epoxidase in ergosterol biosynthesis pathway	291.4	Mycologic: 69.9 Complete: 4.5
Azole	Bifonazole	1% cream	40% urea for 2 to 4 weeks, then bifonazole cream for 6 to 8 weeks (urea as adjunct) or Bifonazole + 40% urea (combination)	Inhibits lanosterol 14α-demethylase in ergosterol biosynthesis pathway	310.4	**Urea as adjunct** Mycologic: 42.6–69 Complete: 27.7 **Combination** Mycologic: 58.3–82.8 Complete: 20.8
	Efinaconazole	10% solution	Once-daily for 48 weeks	Inhibits lanosterol 14α-demethylase in ergosterol biosynthesis pathway	349.39	Mycologic: 53.4–55.2 Complete: 15.8–17.2
	Luliconazole	5% solution	Once-daily for 48 weeks	Inhibits lanosterol 14α-demethylase in ergosterol biosynthesis pathway Inhibition of extracellular protease secretion	354.28	Mycologic: 45.4 Complete: 14.9
	Ketaconazole	Nanoemulgel containing permeation enhancer	TBD	Inhibits lanosterol 14α-demethylase in ergosterol biosynthesis pathway	531.43	TBD
		Ketoconazole-encapsulated cross-linked fluorescent supramolecular nanoparticles	TBD	Inhibits lanosterol 14α-demethylase in ergosterol biosynthesis pathway	531.43	TBD
Benzoxaboroles	Tavaborole	5% solution	Once-daily for 48 weeks	Inhibits fungal proteins synthesis by inhibiting aminoacyl transfer RNA synthetase	151.93	Mycologic: 31.1–35.9 Complete: 6.5–9.1

Other	AN-2718	TBD	Inhibits fungal proteins synthesis by inhibiting aminoacyl transfer RNA synthetase	168.39	TBD
	AR-12 (OSU-03012)	TBD	Inhibits acetyl CoA synthase in the fungal wall, and downregulates host chaperone proteins	460.45	TBD
	Auriclosene (NVC-422)	TBD	Protein inactivation *via* modification of sulfur-containing amino acids	222.09	TBD
	ME-1111	TBD	Inhibits succinate dehydrogenase (complex II) in the mithocondrial electron transport system	202.25	TBD

Note: TBD: to be determined.

Topical Polymer Barriers

A topical polymer barrier for the nail plate has been developed. This drug-free formulation coats the nail plate occluding water and external matter from infiltrating the nail plate structure. The film is applied 5 days a week, removed on the 6th, and restarted the following week. After 6 months, 63% of trial participants had negative mycological cultures.

Device-Based Therapies

Device-based therapy is an expanding area of onychomycosis therapy. Devices can be used to enhance drug delivery, activate topically applied drugs or photothermally kill fungi. Device-based therapy has a number of advantages over traditional onychomycosis therapy because these procedures are primarily conducted in the clinic by trained professionals, reducing the need for patient compliance. Since device-based therapies utilize topical drugs, the risk of systemic interactions and adverse reactions are negligible.

Device-based treatments reduce the need for long-term patient compliance.

Photodynamic Therapy

Photodynamic therapy (PDT) is a non-invasive therapy utilizing visible spectrum light to activate a topically applied photosensitizing agent. Photosensitizers are substances that absorb light energy and transfer it to adjacent molecules, in this case fungi. PDT generates reactive oxygen species and initiates the destruction of cells by necrosis or apoptosis. Molecules approved by the FDA include 5-aminolevulinic acid (ALA) and methylaminolevulate (MAL). ALA and MAL were developed for the treatment of dermal lesions, including actinic keratoses and nonmelanoma skin cancer, but are also be used off-label for the treatment of onychomycosis. In clinical trials using ALA and MAL PDT, the nail plate is typically pre-treated with urea to enhance penetration and aid in photosensitizer uptake. The ALA or MAL is usually applied for 3–5 hours and then treated with a red light device, usually at 630 nm or a spectrum from 570 nm to 670 nm. *In vitro*, methylene blue-mediated photodynamic therapy was fungicidal to *T. rubrum*. In one clinical trial (n = 30), the clinical cure rate was 36.6% at 18 months. In another study (n = 22), the mycologic cure rate was 100%, and the complete cure rates were 63.6% and 100% in patients with severe, and mild to moderate onychomycosis, respectively. Limitations include the pre-treatment with nail avulsion or urea and numerous required sessions for efficacy. In addition, most patients experience pain, requiring breaks in the middle of the treatment.

Iontophoresis

Iontophoresis devices use AN electric current to increase drug uptake into the nail plate. Topical terbinafine in a gel or patch formulation can be applied to the nail plate with electric current to enhance terbinafine transport into the nail plate. The nail plate then acts as a reservoir, releasing terbinafine into the underlying tissue over time, to treat onychomycosis.

There are currently two iontophoresis devices in development. The first is a patch device that is worn overnight with a power pack (two printed batteries of 1.5 V each) and two wired electrodes positioned above and beneath the toe. In a preliminary trial involving 38 toenail onychomycosis patients, those treated with this device showed an 84% mycological cure rate at 12-week follow-up, whereas patients treated with the terbinafine patch formulation alone only showed a 48% mycological cure rate. The second device uses wired electrodes positioned at the hyponychium and proximal nail fold, and involves application of terbinafine gel; this device was assayed using an ex vivo model in human cadaver toes. This model showed the amount of drug in the nail plate after application of iontophoresis was approximately 20 times greater when compared with passive delivery. There were also detectable amounts of terbinafine in the nail bed and matrix, compared with passive treatment, which showed undetectable amounts of the drug in these locations.

Laser Systems

Lasers are attractive options for onychomycosis treatment because they avoid systemic side effects associated with oral therapies, application difficulties, and long-term treatment courses associated with topicals. As opposed to other treatment alternatives, lasers are FDA approved for the temporary increase of clear nail for onychomycosis treatment. Therefore, they are assessed based on aesthetic improvements, instead of complete cure, which precludes meaningful comparisons between laser and drug efficacy. In a review, laser-induced improvement rates were compared to those of oral and topical FDA-approved onychomycosis therapies (using medical endpoints). It was concluded that laser treatments (2 studies) resulted in lower mycologic cure rates (11%) compared to oral and topical alternatives (21 studies) (29%–61%). There are other limitations to laser therapies. Multiple sessions are often required, and durations of treatment may exceed 1 year. Furthermore, costs in the United States are usually high, since laser therapy is not covered under most insurance plans. Patients usually experience significant pain and discomfort during treatment.

> Laser-based treatments are FDA approved for cosmetic improvements and not for complete pathogen eradication.

Lasers exert their antifungal effect based on the principle of selective photothermolysis, in that the conversion of radiant laser energy into heat is confined to targeted chromophores. Thus, laser energy may be preferentially absorbed by fungal pathogens, resulting in photothermal and photomechanical damage that spares surrounding human tissues. There are a number of variables that affect the delivery of laser energy through the nail plate including wavelength, pulse format, spot size, and energy fluence. The wavelength of the laser determines the target chromophores and the specific depth at which they lie. A pulsed beam produces short (ms-ns) burst of laser light energy into the target tissue causing a rapid elevation in temperature, while at the same time allowing for tissue cooling to occur, limiting collateral damage. The shorter the laser pulse, the higher the maximum energy of the pulse. The spot size affects the ease of treating the nail plate; a larger spot size will facilitate better coverage of the nail plate. The energy fluence is a measure of the laser energy delivered by area; in many cases longer pulse durations deliver higher energy fluences, despite having a lower maximum pulse energy.

Nd:YAG Lasers

Commercial Nd:YAG lasers have been approved to treat onychomycosis at 1064 nm. Some studies are also examining the use of 532 nm and 1320 nm wavelengths. Nd:YAG 1064 nm lasers come in three pulse durations; millisecond long pulse lasers, microsecond short pulse lasers, and nanosecond Q-switched lasers. In a study conducted using a Fotona Dynamis long-pulse laser system, 93.5% of patients achieved completely clear nail plates and 100% of participants had a negative mycological culture at a 12–18 month follow-up (four laser treatments).

There have been a number of small open-label studies conducted using short-pulse laser systems including the Nuvolase Pin Pointe Foot Laser, the Cutera Genesis Plus, and the Sciton JOULE Clear Sense laser systems. Follow-up visits were conducted between 6 and 9 months, demonstrating an increase in clear nail growth.

A clinical trial was also conducted with a Q-switched laser. The Light Age Q-Clear laser system resulted in an increase in clear nail in 95% of participants with an average clearance of the affected area of 56%.

Although long-pulsed Nd:YAG is one of the most commonly used laser modalities, there is a lack of clearly specified optimized treatment regimen. Some studies suggest weekly, while others monthly treatments. The total number of sessions ranges from 3 to 8, typically with 2 to 3 passes performed on each visit.

Diode Lasers

Diode lasers have not yet been approved to treat onychomycosis in North America; however, two diode lasers are being investigated for the treatment of onychomycosis. The Noveon laser is a dual wavelength 870 nm and 930 nm device, which has been shown to be fungicidal against *T. rubrum* and *C. albicans in vitro*. Clinical trials with this laser resulted in a mycological cure in 30% of participants and improvements in clear nail growth in 85% of participants. An additional clinical trial with 50 participants enrolled with toenail onychomycosis treated with the 980-nm diode V-Raser laser system for four sessions at 6-week interval has been conducted; results are yet to be published.

Fractional Lasers

Fractional laser technology can maximize the photothermal effects of ablative laser therapy by producing small pores in the nail plate and assisting in drug delivery while minimizing side effects. The optimal number and frequency of treatment sessions and selected parameters have not been established and are thus selected based on physician experience.

Standardized treatment parameters with lasers for onychomycosis are lacking.

A recent systematic review and meta-analysis extracted data from 35 articles, including 5 RCT studies. The overall mycological cure rate for laser treatment was 63.0%. In comparison, the mycological efficacy of itraconazole pulse therapy and continuous terbinafine therapy for the treatment of onychomycosis were 79.6% and 84.8%, respectively. However, laser treatment produced less reported systemic side effects than oral therapy. In addition, the analysis suggested that laser treatment appeared to be more suitable for certain population subgroups, such as children, the elderly and pregnant women. The efficacy of CO_2 laser treatment was found to be slightly higher than that of 1064-nm Nd:YAG laser and the efficacy of CO_2 perforated laser treatment was superior to that of CO_2 fractional laser.

Further research into the efficacy of device-based therapies is required before they can be widely recommended.

Conclusions

The treatment armamentarium for onychomycosis is rapidly expanding. Novel therapies center on topical formulations and device-based options because their adverse effects are limited to the application site, with negligible risks of systemic toxicity and drug interactions. In addition, device-based alternatives have the potential to reduce the need for long-term patient compliance. Laser-based treatments are only considered for cosmetic improvements and not for treatment; therefore, meaningful comparison with oral/topical therapies is challenging. Furthermore, standardized treatment parameters with lasers are lacking. These developments may help to improve the efficacy of onychomycosis treatment in the near future. More research and published data with the newer therapeutic modalities will help determine the efficacy of these modalities in the management of dermatophyte and nondermatophyte onychomycosis.

Abbreviations

TNS	Terbinafine nail solution
MOB-015	Terbinafine 10% nail solution
FDA	Food and Drug Administration
NDM	Nondermatophyte mold
KTZ⊂c-FSMNPs	Ketoconazole-encapsulated cross-linked fluorescent supramolecular nanoparticles
tRNA	Aminoacyl-transfer ribonucleic acid
NVC-422	Auriclosene
PDT	Photodynamic therapy
ALA	5-aminolevulinic acid
MAL	Methylaminolevulate

BIBLIOGRAPHY

Elewski B., Brand S., Degenhardt T., Curelop S., Pollak R., Schotzinger R., et al. (2020) A phase II, randomized, double-blind, placebo-controlled, dose-ranging study to evaluate the efficacy and safety of VT-1161 oral tablets in the treatment of patients with distal and lateral subungual onychomycosis of the toenail. *Br J Dermatol.*

Elewski B.E., Rich P., Pollak R., Pariser D.M., Watanabe S., Senda H., et al. (2013) Efinaconazole 10% solution in the treatment of toenail onychomycosis: two phase III multicenter, randomized, double-blind studies. *J Am Acad Dermatol*; 68(4): 600–608.

Elewski B.E., Aly R., Baldwin S.L., Gonzalez Soto R.F., Rich P., Weisfeld M., et al. (2015) Efficacy and safety of tavaborole topical solution, 5%, a novel boron-based antifungal agent, for the treatment of toenail onychomycosis: results from 2 randomized phase-III studies. *J Am Acad Dermatol*; 73(1): 62–69.

Gupta A.K., Versteeg S.G. (2017) A critical review of improvement rates for laser therapy used to treat toenail onychomycosis. *J Eur Acad Dermatol Venereol*; 31(7): 1111–1118.

Gupta A.K., Surprenant M.S., Kempers S.E., Pariser D.M., Rensfeldt K., Tavakkol A. (2020) Efficacy and safety of topical terbinafine 10% solution (MOB-015) in the treatment of mild-to-moderate distal subungual onychomycosis: a randomized, multi-center, double-blind, vehicle-controlled phase 3 study. *J Am Acad Dermatol.*

Iorizzo M., Arraiz G., Frisenda L., Caserini M., Mailland F., (eds). (2013) *An innovative terbinafine transungual solution (P-3058): dose finding investigation on clinical benefit in patients affected by mild-to moderate toe onychomycosis. American Academy of Dermatology.* 71st Annual Meeting, Fla, Miami Beach.

Kubota-Ishida N., Takei-Masuda N., Kaneda K., Nagira Y., Chikada T., Nomoto M., et al. (2018) In vitro human onychopharmacokinetic and pharmacodynamic analyses of ME1111: a new topical agent for onychomycosis. *Antimicrob Agents Chemother*; 62(1).

Kushwaha A.S., Sharma P., Shivakumar H.N., Rappleye C., Zukiwski A., Proniuk S., et al. (2017) Transungual delivery of AR-12, a novel antifungal drug. *AAPS PharmSciTech*; 18(7): 2702–2705.

Lipner S.R., Scher R.K. (2019) Onychomycosis: Treatment and prevention of recurrence. *J Am Acad Dermatol*; 80(4): 853–867.

Lipner S.R., Scher R.K. (2019) Onychomycosis: Clinical overview and diagnosis. *J Am Acad Dermatol*; 80(4): 835–851.

Ma W., Si C., Kasyanju Carrero L.M., Liu H.F., Yin X.F., Liu J., et al. (2019) Laser treatment for onychomycosis: a systematic review and meta-analysis. *Medicine (Baltimore)*; 98(48): e17948.

Mahtab A., Anwar M., Mallick N., Naz Z., Jain G.K., Ahmad F.J. (2016) Transungual delivery of ketoconazole nanoemulgel for the effective management of onychomycosis. *AAPS PharmSciTech*; 17(6): 1477–1490.

Sigurgeirsson B., van Rossem K., Malahias S., Raterink K. (2013) A phase II, randomized, double-blind, placebo-controlled, parallel group, dose-ranging study to investigate the efficacy and safety of 4 dose regimens of oral albaconazole in patients with distal subungual onychomycosis. *J Am Acad Dermatol*; 69(3): 416–425.

Wang F., Yang P., Choi J.S., Antovski P., Zhu Y., Xu X., et al. (2018) Cross-linked fluorescent supramolecular nanoparticles for intradermal controlled release of antifungal drug-a therapeutic approach for onychomycosis. *ACS Nano*; 12(7): 6851–6859.

Watanabe S., Kishida H., Okubo A. (2017) Efficacy and safety of luliconazole 5% nail solution for the treatment of onychomycosis: a multicenter, double-blind, randomized phase III study. *J Dermatol*; 44(7): 753–759.

5

Lichen planus

Dimitris Rigopoulos

Lichen planus (LP) is a relatively common inflammatory skin disease that lasts from months to years. It usually affects people between the age of 30 and 70 and is slightly more prevalent in women than in men. It affects about 1%–2% of the general population. The name "lichen" refers to the lichen plant which grows on rocks or trees, and "planus" means flat. The exact cause of LP is unknown, but it seems to be triggered by stress, genetics, allergic reactions to medicine, and by viral infections such as hepatitis. Sowden et al. (2006) described a case of LP confined to the nails in a patient with primary biliary cirrhosis.

Lichen planus typically affects the skin, nails, vulva, penis, and mucous membranes including the mouth (Table 5.1). LP affects one or more nails in 1%–15% of the cases. Fingernails are found to be more commonly affected than toenails; however, both can be affected.

Five types of nail LP have been described:

- Typical nail matrix LP (80%)
- Nail bed LP
- Trachyonychia
- Idiopathic atrophy of the nails
- Bullous-erosive LP

Specific Signs of LP

Pterygium

Pterygium is due to the inflammation of the nail matrix and remains adherent to the ventral surface of the nail plate, resulting in a subungual extension of the hyponychium and obliteration of the distal groove. Pterygium is rather rare (<5%) and it usually affects only one nail. It is not related to the duration of the disease (Figure 5.1).

TABLE 5.1

Non-Specific Signs of Nail Lichen Planus

Nail matrix	Nail bed
Thinning of the nail plate	Subungual hyperkeratosis
Longitudinal grooving	Longitudinal erythronychia
Longitudinal melanonychia	Subungual hyperpigmentation
Onychorrhexis	Onycholysis
Distal splitting	
Ridging of the nail plate	
Irregular pitting	

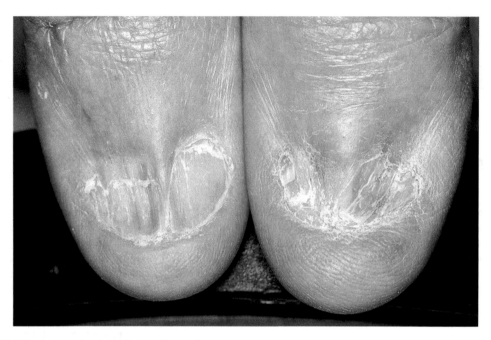

FIGURE 5.1   Pterygium involving two fingernails.

The first fingernails attacked are usually the most severely affected.

Destruction of Nail Matrix and Anonychia

Yellow nail syndrome-like changes may also be a possible sign of nail LP, irrespective of the limbs involved or the number of digits affected. The cause of the yellow color in LP is unknown, but it is speculated that it is due to the relatively poor lymphatic circulation in the lower limbs. Nail LP is most common around the fifth or sixth decades of life. It is not rare in children but probably underestimated (10% of all cases). It mostly affects men. It often presents with atypical clinical features such as 20-nail dystrophy or idiopathic rough nails (Figure 5.2). Skin or mucosal involvement is rarer in children (15%) than in adults with nail LP (25%). Dorsal pterygium formation is rare in children.

Nail bed LP is not so common and it is usually associated with nail plate abnormalities like onycholysis and mild subungual hyperkeratosis. In these cases, nail bed biopsy confirms the diagnosis (Figure 5.3).

Bullous/erosive LP is extremely rare and it is characterized by painful nail erosions (Figure 5.4). It usually affects one or two toenails, and it may be associated with erosive LP elsewhere. Scar formation is usual after treatment.

Nail degloving syndrome, which includes a thimble-shaped nail shedding with the walls of the thimble composed of the skin of the distal digit including the nail plate, a partially sloughed-off nail plate with its surrounding tissue and sparing of the surrounding epidermis of the distal digit, can be caused by, among others, nail lichen planus.

Diagnosis

Clinical features of LP may be difficult to diagnose. A biopsy of the nail is difficult to perform and is rarely an imperative. Histopathologically, LP is characterized by compact orthokeratosis, wedge-shaped hypergranulosis, irregular acanthosis, damage of the basal cell layer, and a band-like inflammatory

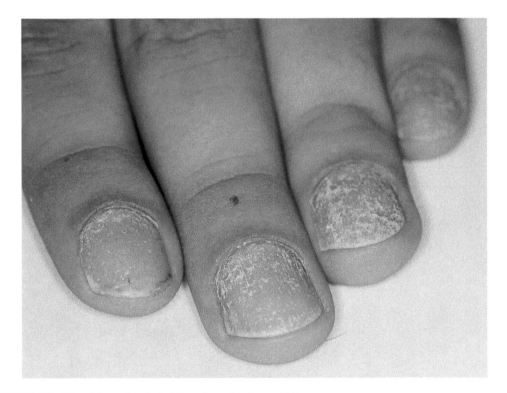

FIGURE 5.2   Idiopathic rough nails in lichen planus (trachyonychia).

infiltrate in the upper dermis. Lymphocytes are the predominant cells making up the infiltrate, along with a few macrophages, eosinophils, and plasma cells. In addition, melanophages are often found in the upper dermis adjacent to the damaged basal cells. Presence of Civatte bodies (also known as colloid bodies and hyaline bodies), represents degenerated, apoptotic keratinocytes.

Mottled erythema of the lunula can be evident, but it is not a specific sign for nail lichen planus. Differential diagnosis includes nail changes caused by graft-vs-host disease, lichenoid drug reactions, nail scarring after Stevens–Johnson syndrome, nail matrix trauma, and lupus erythematosus.

Treatment

Since the etiology of the disease is unknown, treatment is symptomatic and usually anti-inflammatory.

Ungual LP can range from minor nail dystrophy to anonychia. Therefore, treatment should be implemented immediately to avoid permanent deformity or total nail loss. This condition is generally unresponsive to most treatments.

Do not treat dorsal pterygium: it is not reversible! Do not treat trachyonychia: it cures spontaneously!

Topical steroids applied to the involved sites appear to be effective in some cases. Use with occlusive dressing seems to have better results. Triamcinolone acetonide, 0.5 mg/kg im every 30 days, for 3–6 months and then tapered off – is the treatment of choice. Intralesional injection of corticosteroids – triamcinolone acetonide 0.5–0.1 mg/nail every 2 months – can also be used, but is quite a painful

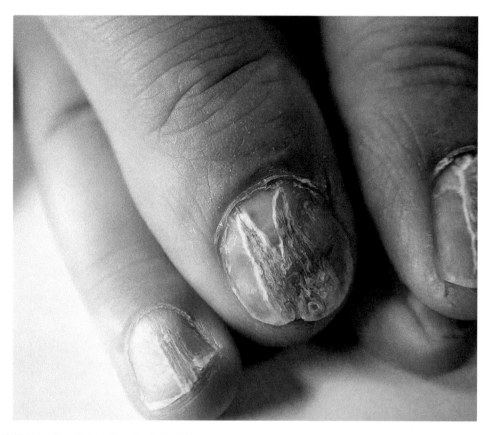

FIGURE 5.3   Superficial nail dystrophy in lichen planus.

therapy. Oral prednisone 0.5 mg/kg for 3 weeks has been successful in some cases. Acitretin can be considered as monotherapy or in combination with topical steroids.

Mostafa (1989) demonstrated a marked improvement of nail LP with chloroquine phosphate 250 mg twice daily; clearance was noted after 30 weeks. However, 10 weeks after discontinuation of therapy, nail lesions recurred.

In 2010, Ujiie and others published five cases of nail LP, treated with Tacrolimus ointment 0.1%, twice a day, with great improvement after 6 months, with no adverse reactions reported.

Alitretinoin – 30 mg once a day, for the first 3 months and then reduced to 10 mg daily to maintain long-term efficacy, may be useful.

Azathioprine – 100 mg daily may be used in association with systemic steroids, in non-responder patients, in order to increase response to therapy.

Etretinate – 0.3–0.4 mg/kg/day may be used in patients non-respondent to systemic steroids, alone or in combination with topical steroids.

Low-dose methotrexate therapy (10–20 mg once-weekly subcutaneously) in two patients was reported to produce significant improvement after a few weeks.

Case reports of cyclosporine have shown improvement within 2 months; however, complications of hypertension limited the duration of therapy.

Monotherapy with etanercept, a TNF-alpha inhibitor, was reported in a case study to be efficacious after 6–9 months of treatment in a patient who had failed other therapies.

Controlled keratolysis of the nail plate with application of 70% glycolic acid can be a promising treatment with cosmetically pleasing results.

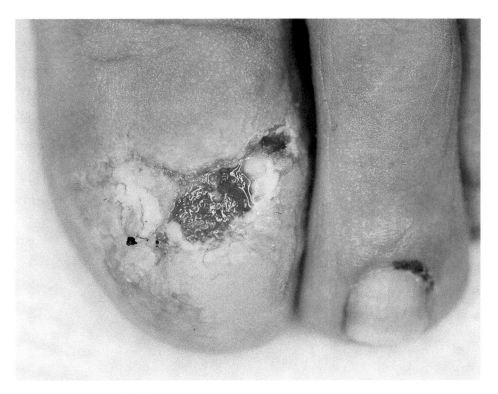

FIGURE 5.4   Erosive ulcerated lichen planus.

- Treat before pterygium formation.
- Children under the age of 12 do not need treatment, unless pterygium has started to appear.
- Patients who do not respond to systemic steroids will not improve with the addition of either azathioprine or systemic retinoids.

- About 50% of patients will not be cured, despite any treatment.
- There is anecdotal evidence for a beneficial response following a short course of topically applied 5% 5-FU.
- Biotin: 2.5 mg daily in young children and 7.5–10 mg in adults has been advised for 6 months.

FURTHER READING

Baran R., Perrin C. (2008) Nail degloving, a polyetiologic condition with three main patterns: a new syndrome. *JAAD*; 58: 232–237.

Banga G. and Patel K. (2014 Oct–Dec) Glycolic acid peels for nail rejuvenation. *J Cutan Aesthet Surg*; 7(4): 198–201.

Goettmann S., Zaraa I., Moulonguet I. (2012) Nail lichen planus: epidemiological, clinical, pathological, therapeutic and prognosis study of 67 cases. *JEADV*; 26(10):1304–1309.

Gordon K. A., Vega J. M., Tosti A. (2011) Trachyonychia: a comprehensive review. *Indian J Dermato lVenereol Leprol*; 77:640–645.

McClanahan D. R., English J. C. 3rd (2018 Aug). Therapeutics for Adult Nail Psoriasis and Nail Lichen Planus: A Guide for Clinicians. *Am J Clin Dermatol*.; 19(4):559–584.

Mostafa W. Z. 1989 Lichen planus of the nail: treatment with antimalarials. *JAAD*; 20(2 pt 1): 289–290.

Piraccini B. M., Saccani E., Starace M., et al. (2010) Nail lichen planus: response to treatment and long term follow-up. *Eur J Dermatol*; 20:489–496.

Sehgal V. N. (2007) Twenty nail dystrophy trachyonychia: an overview. *J Dermatol*; 34:361–366.

Sowden J. M., Cartwright P. H., Green J. R., et al. (2006) Isolated lichen planus of the nails associated with primary biliary cirrhosis. *Br J Dermatol*; 121:659–662.

Tosti A., Piraccini B. M., Cambiaghi S., et al. (2001) Nail lichen planus in children clinical features, response to treatment, and long-term follow-up. *Arch Dermatol*; 137:1027–1032.

Ujiie H., Shibaki A., Akiyama M., et al. (2010) Successful treatment of nail lichen planus with topical tacrolimus. *Acta Derm Venereol*; 90:218–219.

6

Onychotillomania (onychophagia, habit tic, median canaliform onychodystrophy)

Dimitris Rigopoulos

These conditions are described together as in some cases overlapping has been described.

Onychotillomania is defined as a chronic and repetitive manifestation, characterized by the compulsive or irresistible urge of patients to sting parts of the nail apparatus. This can be done by using patient's hands or nails, but practically any tool can used like knifes, scissors, and toothpicks. Depression and hypochondrial delusions have been described in patients with onychotillomania. It is rather uncommon (affecting not more than 0.9% of the population) and a likely underreported or frequently misdiagnosed condition. Shortening distortion or even complete extraction of the nail plate, as well as onychoatrophy, macrolunula, transverse grooves, patchy, or generalized rough areas or thinning of the nail plate, may be present (Figures 6.1, 6.2). Activation of nail matrix melanocytes, due to continues trauma, can result in longitudinal melanonychia, which can persist for months or even years, despite the cessation of nail picking (Figure 6.3). Multiple fissures, cuts, or even ulcerations on the

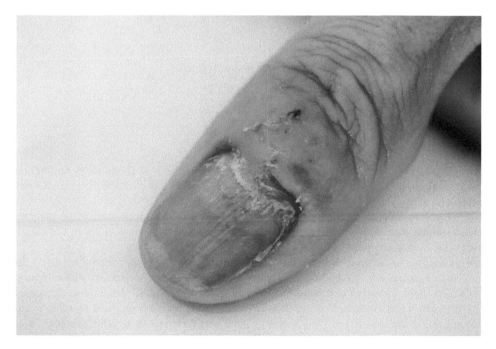

FIGURE 6.1 Onychoatrophy, macrolunula, transverse grooves, and patchy or generalized rough areas of the nail plate may be indications of onychotillomania.

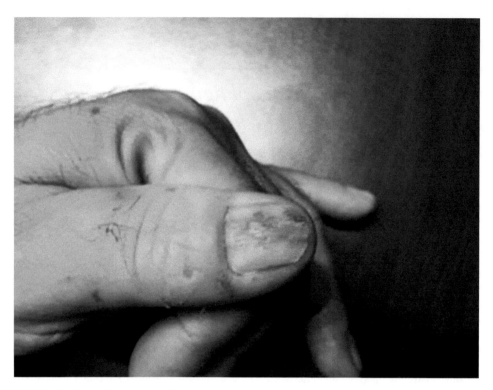

FIGURE 6.2   Onychoatrophy, macrolunula, transverse grooves, and patchy or generalized rough areas of the mnail plate may be indications of onychotillomania.

surrounding tissues may also be seen (Figure 6.4). The wide clinical presentations of this entity can masquerade several inflammatory disorders.

Onychotillomania is 50 times less frequent than onychophagia.

Diagnosis

Diagnosis is based on clinical criteria, while dermoscopy could be helpful. Dermoscopy findings include scales, absence of the nail plate, wavy lines, hemorrhages, speckled dots, melanonychia, and nail bed pigmentation.

Bacterial and viral infections, resulting in paronychia and herpetic whitlow, are some of the complications associated with the disease. In the literature, there is one case report with onychotillomania of the toenails and foot cellulitis as a complication.

Onychophagia is considered as the habit of biting nails, frequently encountered between children (37% of the cases are seen in children 2–13 years old), which can be associated with different phycological conditions (attention deficit hyperactivity disorder, oppositional defiant disorder, separation anxiety disorder, major depressive disorders), especially when it is accompanied by other symptoms of the underlying disease. It can persist in adulthood and can lead to onychodystrophy, which in some cases can be severe (Figure 6.5). It is usually limited to fingernails, and it not infrequent for this condition to be found in members of the same family. Oral and dental problems can be seen in some cases, such as dental crowding, rotations, or malocclusion.

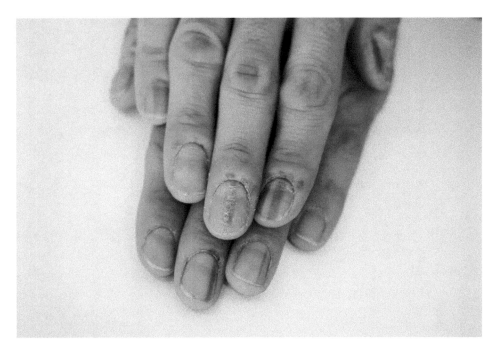

FIGURE 6.3   Longitudinal melanonychia.

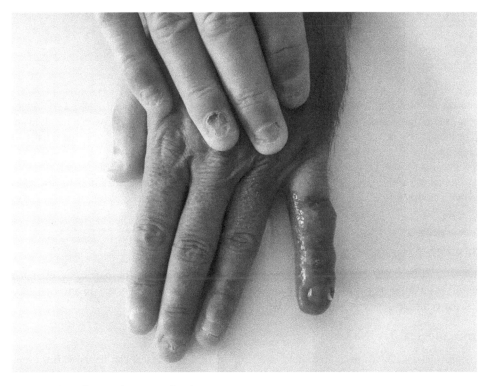

FIGURE 6.4   Ulcerations on the surrounding tissues.

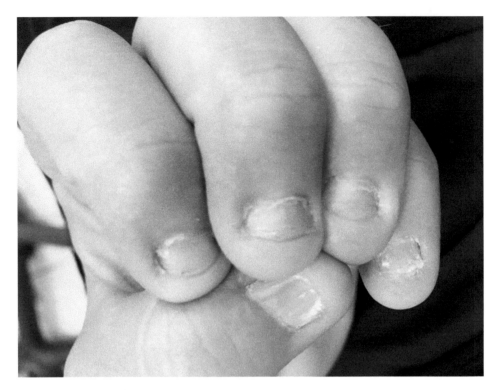

FIGURE 6.5   Severe onychodystrophy.

Children with onychophagia are usually bullied by their friends.

Habit-tic deformity is a nail dystrophy found usually on both thumbnails, and very seldom on toenails. Patients are usually unaware of doing such a repetitive trauma of the proximal nail fold and as a result of the underlying nail matrix. Nails in such a condition are described as "washboard nails" due to their resemblance to a washboard (Figure 6.6).

Median canaliform onychodystrophy is an idiopathic rare nail plate entity, which can also result from continues picking of the cuticular part of the nail fold. It has also been described in patients undergoing isotretinoin treatment.

Treatment

Treatment of all three above mentioned disorders is still rather difficult and, in some cases, disappointing. One of the main difficulties is to convince patients for their behavioral disturbance. In any case, treatment aims at the complete cessation of these habits.

Pharmacological Treatment

Anti depressants, sedatives or antipsychotic drugs, in more severe cases, can be used. But even then, these are only in few cases effective, especially when patients have co existent depression or psychosis.

In a recent meta-analysis of 11 randomized controlled review studies, no benefit was shown to pharmacotherapy over placebo for treating skin-picking disorders.

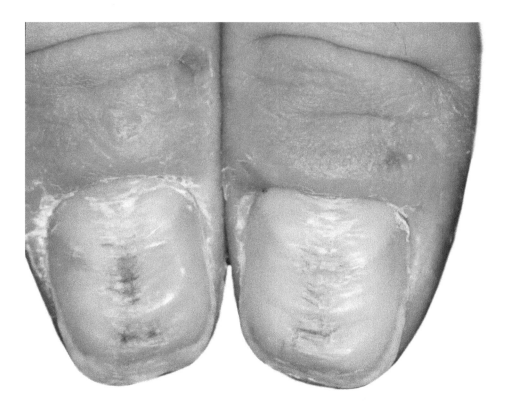

FIGURE 6.6 Thickening of the PNF and torn "hang nails."

N-acetylcysteine, a thiol compound, has among other anti-inflammatory, neurotransmission modulation activity and antiproliferative effects. It has been used in cases of onychophagia at a dose of 200–800 mg/day in children and adolescents, and it showed that it increased the rate of the nail length significantly more than the placebo, after only 1 month of treatment, but not after 2 months.

Biotin (a water soluble vitamin B) has been used to treat habit tic deformity of the nail, in a dosage of 6000 mcg/day, in a multivitamin containing drug, in two patients. Results were considered excellent, with complete recovery after 4 months of treatment. Biotin is considered to increase strength and hardness of the nail plate. We should take into account the rare risk of interference of Biotin with laboratory tests and the mimic Graves' disease. Skin rashes, digestive upset, problems with insulin release, and kidney's pathology have also been reported with high doses of this drug.

Topical tacrolimus ointment was applied in one patient with median canaliform onychodystrophy, for 4 months, once a day, with good results. The exact effect is obscure, but it is probably based on the anti-inflammatory effect of the drug.

Non-Pharmacological Treatment

Gentle massage of the nail, from the matrix area to the free edge, with a bland ointment, three times/day, has been reported to be helpful in some cases. Physical barriers, like wrapping with bandages and tapes or using gloves that occlude the area of the nails that are affected, have also been used. Unpleasant-flavored topical agents, including capsicum, neem oil and denatonium benzoate (that give a bitter taste), can be used alternatively.

Behavioral modification perhaps is the best approach in these patients.

Cyanoacrylate adhesives, known as "super glue," applied one to two times a week in order to create an occlusion area overlying the cuticle, has been used with good results after 4–6 months. Susceptible patients must be careful as allergic contact dermatitis may appear.

Auricular acupressure has also been used in children with nail biting with great improvement, by reducing anxiety.

Intraoral fixed habit-breaker device and a stainless steel twisted round wire bonded from canine to canine have been used, with good results, in patients with onychophagia.

FURTHER READING

Adil M, Amin S, Mohtashim M. 2018 Nacetylcysteine in dermatology. *IJDVL* (6): 652–659.

Haltch P, Scher R, Lipner S. 2017 Onychotillomania: diagnosis and management. *Am J Clin Dermatol*; 18(6): 763–770.

Rieder E, Tosti A. 2016 Onychotillomania: an underrecognized disorder. *JAAD*; 75(6): 1245–1250.

Sidiropoulou P, Sgouros D, Theodoropoulos K, et al. 2019 A chameleon like disorder: case report and review of literature. *SAD*; 5: 104–107.

Singal A, Daulatabad D. 2017 Nail tic disorders: manifestations, pathogenesis and management. *IJDVL*.; 83(1): 19–26.

Sun D, Reziwan K, Wang J, et al. 2018 Auricular acupressure improves habit reversal treatment for nail biting. *The J of Alternative medicine*.; 25:1–7.

7

Eczema

Dimitris Rigopoulos
Robert Baran

The nail apparatus is extremely sensitive to allergic or irritant hazards and eczema in this region is frequent. Atopic dermatitis is an important factor for hand eczema. The high frequency of hand eczema in women, in comparison with men is caused by environmental and not genetic factors. The appearance of the nail depends on the extend of the severity of the disorder and the location of the primary pathology in the nail bed, matrix, or supporting periungual tissues (Silverman 2017).

> The high frequency of hand eczema in women is caused by environmental factors.

Atopic dermatitis is the most prevalent among primary skin diseases in children. Pruritus, a major criterion for diagnosis and infection, with *Staphylococcus aureus*, a major complication, are directly responsible for nail diseases in this disorder. Fingernail plates of atopic children with chronic disease may be shiny and buffed from constant rubbing (Richert and André 2011). Disruption of the cuticle and inflammation of the matrix during intense atopic flares may result in wavy irregular repetitive transverse grooves or varying size of length. Bacterial paronychia can develop from overt infection or heavy colonization with *S. aureus* or *Streptococcus pyogenes*. One should be alert for a distinctive presentation of Staph infection that may be associated with underlying osteomyelitis of the distal phalanx.

> Bacterial paronychia may develop.

These patients have one or more black, triangular-shaped infarct-like macules under the distal free edge of the nail. These may be associated with painful dactylitis. If there is no underlying bone infection present, antiseptic washes with chlorhexidine, along with topical antimicrobial therapy, may be sufficient. Contact allergy is confirmed as a significant risk for hand eczema and related to its strength. Ingredients in nail care products may lead to allergic and/or irritant contact dermatitis. The latter can result in nail plate yellowing, nail dystrophy and cuticle disruption. Allergic contact dermatitis to nail polish has been reported to most commonly present as ectopic dermatitis as allergens are transferred by direct contact from partially dried polish.

So far, "no single classification of hand eczema is completely satisfactory," but that of Lachapelle (2014) – into exogenous (contact dermatitis), endogenous (eczema), and exogenous and/or endogenous (dermatitis) – is helpful.

See also Figure 7.1 and Table 7.1.

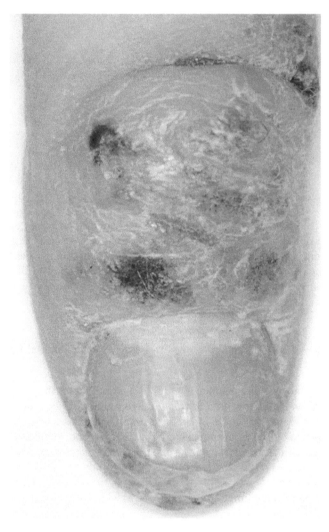

FIGURE 7.1   Infected contact dermatitis in a housewife.

Treatment

Application of paraben-free topical corticosteroids three times daily to the surrounding soft tissues is considered as the first line therapy in the treatment of eczema. The choice of steroid potency is influenced by factors such as eczema severity and morphology. Drug delivery is enhanced with an ointment vehicle as well as with occlusion. In addition, water soaks for 20 mn prior to steroid application, appear to give superior results improving pruritus and xerosis (Lodén et al. 2012). Chronic dermatitis may be improved with ciclosporin and even alitretinoin. The effectiveness of topical calcineurin inhibitors, such as pimecrolimus or tacrolimus used in the treatment of ectopic dermatitis, prevents some complications of corticosteroids, such as "disappearing digit" (see Chapter 20).

The management of allergic contact dermatitis (ACD) is based on the identification of the offending allergen, avoidance of exposure, use of safe alternatives, and treatment of symptoms, although corticosteroids remain the first choice of therapy for many clinicians, the chronic nature of the disease

TABLE 7.1

Clinical Reaction Patterns and Their Origin

Proximal nail matrix	

- Pitting (small depressions on the dorsum of the plate)
- Beau's lines and transverse grooving
- Trachyonychia (rough nails due to excessive ridging)
- Onychomadesis (detachment of the nail in its proximal portion)
- Nail shedding (loss of fingernail due to persistent contact dermatitis in an artificial gel nail designer is rarely reported)

Distal matrix

- Leukonychia

Nail bed and hyponychium

- Onycholysis (distal and/or lateral detachment of the nail plate

Paronychium

- Paronychial involvement (LE-like erythema and periungual telangiectasia among coffee plantation workers)
- When eczema occurs on the proximal and lateral nail folds, erythema, edema, and loss of the cuticle can result, characteristic of a chronic paronychia. The potential space between the proximal nail fold and the nail plate harbors moisture and Candida yeast. Eczema will affect the most proximal part of the matrix if it involves the proximal nail fold.

Surrounding tissue

- Changes in the surrounding tissue (pulpitis, fissures)

Surrounding contour

- Changes in the texture and contour of the nail plate, onychauxis, worn-down nail plate (usure des ongles), brittle nails, koilonychias (in Ladakh, after exposure to cold, wet mud)

Underlying bone

- Distal bony phalanx anomalies (they are mainly responsible for shape of the nail, pseudo-acro-osteolysis)

Source: From Lachapelle 2014. With permission.

and the many side effects associated with corticosteroids remain a major obstacle in their long-term use.

Emerging biologic therapies with licensed indications for other eczematous and immuno-inflammatory skin conditions, mainly monoclonal antibodies inhibiting tumor necrosis factor alpha, interleukin 12 (IL-12), IL-17, IL-23, IL-4, and immunoglobulin E (IgE), may have a place in the treatment of recalcitrant cases of ACD. These newer agents offer major promises in the treatment of contact dermatitis by targeting specific mediators or pathways of inflammation" (from Bhatia 2020, with permission).

When systemic antibiotics are necessary, probiotics and prebiotics present beneficial effects on allergic diseases (Karadag 2020).

Preventive measures are also those observed in case of nail fragility, but above all one must follow a very strict protocol of wearing two pairs of gloves: cotton beneath vinyl gloves.

Protective gloves should also be worn by sensitized beauticians. Double nitrile gloves provide up 60 minutes of protection, but thicker, 4H plastic polymer gloves offer complete protection (Warshaw 2020).

BIBLIOGRAPHY

Baran R., (2014) Nail alterations in hand eczema in: Alikahn A., Lachapelle J. M., Maibach H. *Textbook of Hand Eczema*, Springer.

Bhatia J., Sarin A., Wollina U. et al. (2020) Review of biologics in allergic contact dermatitis. *Contact dermatitis*; 1–3.

Dolma T., Norboo T., Yayha M. et al. (1990), Seasonal koilonychia in Ladakh. *Contact Dermatitis.* 22(2): 78–80.

Karadag A. S., Kayiran M. A., Parish L. C. (2020) Skin med probiotics and prebotics. *The good germs: A dermatologic perspective*; 18: 10–13.

Lachapelle J. M., (2014) Clinical subtypes and categorization of hand eczema: an overview in: Alikahn A., Lachapelle J. M., Maibach H. *Textbook of Hand Eczema*, Springer.

Lodén M., Wirén K., Smerud K. T., et al. (2012) The effect of the corticosteroid cream and a barrier-strengthening moisturizer in hand eczema. A double-blind, randomized, prospective, parallel group clinical trial. *JEADV*; 26: 597–601.

Richert B., André J. (2011) Nail disorders in children: diagnosis and management. *Am J Clin Dermatol*; 12: 101–112.

Silverman R. (2017) in: Baran R., Hadj Rabia S., Silverman R. *Pediatric nail disorders; chap 8*. CRC Press.

Warshaw E. M. et al. (2020) Contact dermatitis associated with nail care products: Retrospective analysis of North American Contact Dermatitis Group Data, 2001–2016. *Dermatitis*; 31: 191–201.

8

Acrodermatitis continua of Hallopeau

Dimitris Rigopoulos

This disease was first introduced in 1890 by Hallopeau and termed "pyodermite vegetante." It is a disease with etiology and pathomechanism still unknown, but despite this fact, it is considered by many authors to be a variant of pustular psoriasis with a chronic relapsing course.

Approximately 30% of the patients with palmoplantar pustulosis have nail involvement. Continuous pustulation causes nail destruction and atrophy of the distal phalanxes.

Pustules

These are small sterile pustules, located around the nail folds and under the nail plate, starting on one or two fingers or less, often on the toes, and they are surrounded by a hyperemic area (Figure 8.1).

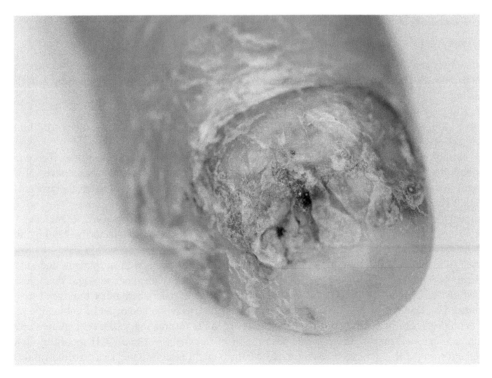

FIGURE 8.1   Acrodermatitis continua.

TABLE 8.1

Signs of Acrodermatitis

Pustules
Onychodystrophy
Paronychia
Onycholysis
Osteolysis of the distal phalanges of the fingers and toes
Loss of the nail

Continuous pustulation of the nail bed and nail matrix may lead to nail destruction, atrophy of the distal phalanx followed by total destruction of the nail bed, and severe onychodystrophy.

Onycholysis

This is due to the accumulation of purulent-appearing material and scales that form thick exudating masses under the nail.

Young patients including children with one finger or toe impacted are the individuals affected by the disease.

Treatment

Treatment for acrodermatitis continua of Hallopeau is known to be more difficult than for other chronic pustular diseases and rather disappointing as most of the drugs used do not achieve any long-lasting remission.

First-line systemic therapy for ACH includes acitretin. In a dosage of 0.5 mg/kg/day, it seems to be effective after 4–6 months of treatment. Acitretin has also been combined with calcipotriol ointment with impressive improvement in one case.

Second-line systemic therapy involves the use of cyclosporine and biologic agents. A recent review described that most of the biological therapies available for treating plaque psoriasis have shown response in the management of ACH as well, although higher doses and combination therapy are often required. The humanized anti-TNF-alpha monoclonal antibody infliximab, 3 mg/kg, was given intravenously. After 4 months, a substantial improvement of the lesions was observed. Etanercept 50 mg twice a week and methotrexate 10 mg/week seems to control the disease satisfactorily. Adalimumab, in combination with acitretin 50 mg/day, proved to be efficacious in dealing with a case of refractory disease. Adalimumab was also used as monotherapy in three patients with a dramatic and sustained response. The previous treatment of two of the three had failed with other biologic therapies. This showed that adalimumab can be effective in acrodermatitis continua, where other biological treatment has failed. Ustekinumab has been reported to be effective both as monotherapy and combination therapy with acitretin. There have also been published cases of ACH responding to the IL-17A inhibitors secukinumab and ixekizumab. There is one case report of treatment-resistant ACH reporting rapid improvement with the IL-1 inhibitor, anakinra. Brodalumab might be considered as a possible valid choice for the management of recalcitrant ACH, with two reported cases in the literature. Apremilast may be useful as the second-line treatment of ACH that is recalcitrant to conventional therapeutic modalities, as three case reports have demonstrated.

Targeted ultraviolet B 311 nm phototherapy was reported to control the disease in one case.

Calcipotriol ointment was applied twice a day and suppressed almost completely the formation of new pustules in one patient.

Excellent response to the combination of thalidomide and ultraviolet was reported in an infant with the disease.

One patient was treated with topical 8-methoxypsoralen without occlusion, plus local narrow band ultraviolet B phototherapy.

Oral tetracycline with betamethasone cream under occlusion appeared to be very effective in treating the disease.

Tacrolimus ointment 0.1% twice a day alone as monotherapy, under occlusion with kitchen foil or in combination with calcipotriol ointment, has proved successful in dealing with acrodermatitis continua.

Disease localized on both great toes, was treated with excellent results with an ointment containing both calcipotriol and betamethasone dipropionate.

Dapsone at a dosage of 200 mg/day was used with excellent results after 4 weeks.

Treat the patient, NOT the disease.

FURTHER READING

Balato N., Gallo L., Balato A., et al. (2009) Acrodermatitis continua of Hallopeau responding to efalizumab therapy. *J Eur Acad Dermatol Venereol*; 23: 1329–1330.

Bordignon M., Zattra E., Albertin C., et al. (2010) Successful treatment of a 9-year-old boy affected by acrodermatitis continua of Hallopeau with targeted ultraviolet B narrow-band phototherapy. *Photodermatol Photoimmunol Photomed*; 26: 41–43.

Brunasso A. M., Lo Scocco G., Massone C. (2008) Recalcitrant acrodermatitis continua of hallopeau treated with calcitriol and tacrolimus 0.1% topical treatment. *J Eur Acad Dermatol Venereol*; 22: 1272–1273.

Caputo F., Parro S., Zoli G. (2011) Adalimumab for a co-existing clinical condition of Crohn's disease and acrodermatitis continua of Hallopeau. *J Crohns Colitis*; 5: 649.

Kurihara Y., Nakano K., Eto A., Furue M. (2019 Oct) Successful treatment of acrodermatitis continua of Hallopeau with apremilast. *J Dermatol*; 46(10): e370–e371.

Maliyar K., Crowley E. L., Rodriguez-Bolanos F., et al. (2019 Jul/Aug) The use of biologic therapy in the treatment of acrodermatitis continua of Hallopeau: a review. *Journal of Cutaneous Medicine and Surgery*; 23(4): 428–435

Milani-Nejad N., Kaffenberger J. (2019) Treatment of recalcitrant acrodermatitis continua of Hallopeau with brodalumab. *J Drugs Dermatol*; 18: 1047.

Passante M., Dastoli S., Nisticò S. P., et al. Effectiveness of brodalumab in acrodermatitis continua of Hallopeau: a case report. *Dermatologic Therapy*. Jan; 33(1): e13170

Puig L., Barco D., Vilarrasa E., et al. (2010) Treatment of acrodermatitis continua of Hallopeau with TNF-blocking agents: case report and review. *Dermatology*; 220: 154–158.

Rubio C., Martin M. A., Arranz Sánchez D. M., et al. (2009) Excellent and prolonged response to infliximab in a case of recalcitrant acrodermatitis continua of Hallopeau. *J Eur Acad Dermatol Venereol*; 23: 707–708.

Ryan C., Collins P., Kirby B., et al. (2009) Treatment of acrodermatitis continua of Hallopeau with adalimumab. *Br J Dermatol*; 160: 203–205.

Sehgal V. N., Verma P., Sharma S., et al. (2011) Acrodermatitis continua of Hallopeau: evolution of treatment options. *Int J Dermatol*; 50: 1195–1211.

Silpa-archa N., Wongpraparut C. (2011) A recalcitrant acrodermatitis continua of Hallopeau successfully treated with etanercept. *J Med Assoc Thai*; 94: 1154–1157.

Sotiriadis D., Patsatsi A., Sotiriou E., et al. (2007) Acrodermatitis continua of Hallopeau on toes successfully treated with a two-compound product containing calcipotriol and betamethasone dipropionate. *J Dermatol Treat*; 18: 315–318.

9

Herpes simplex (herpetic whitlow, herpetic paronychia)

Dimitris Rigopoulos

Pathogen: Herpes Simplex Type I or II

This infection can be found in any age group. However, it is most common in children who suck their thumbs and in healthcare providers who are exposed to patients' oral mucosa without glove protection. This diagnosis is of particular importance due to its close similarity to paronychia and its drastically differing treatment. It is classically self-limited and usually resolves in 2–4 weeks for primary infection. The patient should therefore be counseled that the chance of recurrence is about 30%–50%.

Usually one fingernail (forefinger or thumb) is affected (there is only one case in the literature of a patient with herpes simplex infection on all ten fingernails).

Vesicles

Vesicles appear after an inoculation period of 3–10 days. They may precede or follow erythema and pain. They may coalesce and a yellowish honeycomb appearance of the lesions may be evident. Subungual hemorrhage is not rare. Superinfections with *Staphylococci* spp. and *Streptococci* spp. may occur. Sometimes vesicles are less apparent and ulcerations may be seen (Figure 9.1).

Pain

The sensation is usually described as burning pain and it is intense. It is out of proportion to the skin lesions and helps differential diagnosis of herpetic whitlow from acute bacterial paronychia.

TABLE 9.1

Signs of Herpes Simplex

Erythema
Vesicle formation
Pain
Paronychia
Small subungual hematoma

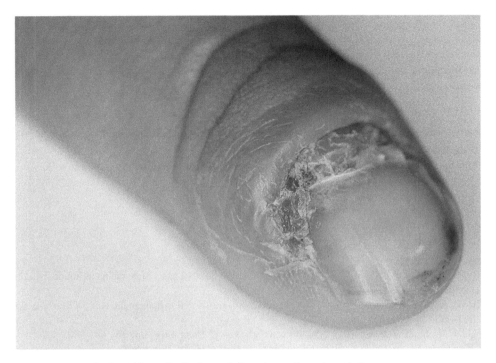

FIGURE 9.1 Herpes simplex with proximal subungual ulcerations and onychomadesis.

Paronychia

It has the characteristics of acute paronychia with erythema, swelling, and the aforementioned pain. Healing takes place over 2–3 weeks.

Diagnosis

Tzanck smear, culture, or rapid immunofluorescence will establish the diagnosis.

Blistering distal dactylitis is a distinct clinical entity manifested by a superficial blistering lesions over the anterior fat pad of the distal portion of a finger or thumb. BDD presents as tense, non-tender bullae due to beta-hemolytic streptococcal skin infection. This disease appears almost exclusively in 2–16 year olds, but cases in adults have been reported. The increasing incidence in isolation of Staphylococcus from cases of BDD suggests a change in pathogenic patterns. These bacterial pathogens can be distinguished only by Gram stain and culture.

Treatment

Herpetic whitlow is highly contagious up to 7 days after the vesicles are healed, so avoidance of close contacts should be counseled. Medical personnel should be vigilant as latex gloves may only decrease transmission.

While there are few studies specific to herpetic whitlow, antivirals have been shown to shorten the duration of symptoms by up to 4 days in one study. Data is especially favorable if the antiviral is started within 48 hours of onset of symptoms. However, the role of antiviral agents is still being debated but should be considered in immunocompromised patients, who may develop disseminated disease. Treatment agents include topical acyclovir and systemic valacyclovir or famciclovir for more severe recalcitrant cases. If recurrent forms are preceded by burning or itching, one tablet Acyclovir 800 may prevent the flare, if taken immediately (within the hour following the first signs).

Surgical drainage does not provide added comfort and may increase the risk for superinfections. Large vesicles may be opened to ease discomfort, particularly if they are located in the nail matrix area, since a theoretical risk of causing permanent deformities does exist.

Recurrent forms of the disease might need treatment with antivirals for 6–12 months (suppressive treatment).

- Individuals with oral infection may inoculate themselves if they are nail biters or finger suckers.
- Involvement of toes has been reported but is rare.
- Appropriate patient education, treatment of secondary bacterial infections and close follow-up is all that is required in minor cases.

FURTHER READING

Murthy S. C., Shetty S. (2011) Herpetic whitlow. *Indian Pediatr*; 48: 665.

Rerucha C. M., Ewing J. T., Oppenlander K. E., Cowan W. C. (2019 Feb 15) Acute hand infections. *Am Fam Physician*; 99(4): 228–236.

Richert B., André J. (2011) Nail disorders in children: Diagnosis and management. *Am J Clin Dermatol*; 12: 101–112.

Rubright J. H., Shafritz A. B. (2011) The herpetic whitlow. *J Hand Surg Am*; 36: 340–342.

Shoji K., Saitoh A. (2018 Feb 8) Herpetic whitlow. *N Engl J Med*; 378(6): 563.

Wu I. B., Schwartz R. A. (2007) Herpetic whitlow. *Cutis*; 79: 193–196.

Zemtsov A., Veitschegger M. (1992) *Staphylococcus aureus*-induced blistering. *J Am Acad Dermatol*; 26: 784–785.

10

Acute paronychia

Dimitris Rigopoulos

The most common cause of acute paronychia is direct or indirect trauma to the cuticle or the nail fold. Such trauma may be relatively minor, resulting from ordinary events, such as dishwashing, injury from a splinter or thorn, onychophagia (nail biting), biting or picking at a hangnail, finger sucking, ingrown nail, manicure procedures (trimming or pushing back the cuticles), artificial nail application, or other nail manipulation. Such trauma enables bacterial inoculation of the nail and subsequent infection. The most common causative pathogen is *Staphylococcus aureus*, although *Streptococcus pyogenes*, *Pseudomonas pyocyanea*, and *Proteus vulgaris* can also cause paronychia. In patients with exposure to oral flora, other anaerobic Gram-negative bacteria may also be involved. Acute paronychia can also develop as a complication of an episode of chronic paronychia. Acute paronychia can also occur as a manifestation of other disorders affecting the digits, such as pemphigus vulgaris, lichen planus, psoriasis, acrodermatitis enteropathica, diabetes mellitus, drugs (acitretin, indinavir), or tumors (Bowen's disease, keratoacanthoma).

In patients with acute paronychia only one nail is typically involved.

TABLE 10.1

Signs of Acute Paronychia

Erythema
Edema
Discomfort
Tenderness
Pus

Erythema

Erythema of the proximal and lateral nail folds usually appears 2–5 days after the trauma. If the infection is left untreated it may evolve into a subungual abscess, with pain and inflammation of the nail matrix. As a consequence, transient or permanent dystrophy of the nail plate may occur (Figure 10.1).

Pus

Pus formation can proximally separate the nail from its underlying attachment, causing elevation of the nail plate.

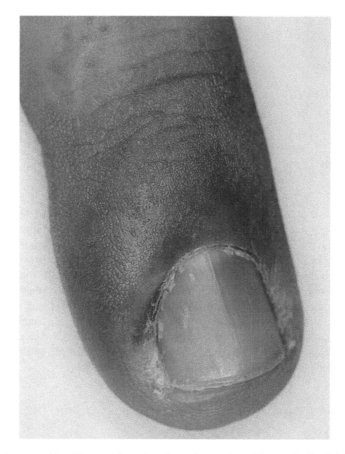

FIGURE 10.1   Acute paronychia with recent formation of pustular reaction of the proximal nail fold.

Recurrent acute paronychia may evolve into chronic paronychia.

Diagnosis

The diagnosis of acute paronychia is based on a history of minor trauma and findings on physical examination of nail folds.

The digital pressure test may be helpful in the early stages of infection when there is doubt about the presence or extent of an abscess. The test is performed by having the patient oppose the thumb and affected finger, thereby applying light pressure to the distal volar aspect of the affected digit. The increase in pressure within the nail fold (particularly in the abscess cavity) causes blanching of the overlying skin and clear demarcation of the abscess. In patients with severe infection or abscess, a specimen should be obtained to identify the responsible pathogen and to rule out methicillin-resistant *S. aureus* (MRSA) infection.

Treatment

Treatment of acute paronychia is determined by the degree of inflammation. If an abscess has not formed, the use of warm water compresses and soaking the affected digit in Burow's solution (i.e., aluminum acetate), vinegar (acetic acid), or chlorhexidine may be effective. Acetaminophen or a nonsteroidal anti-inflammatory drug should be considered for symptomatic relief. Mild cases may be treated with an antibiotic cream (e.g., mupirocin, gentamicin, bacitracin/neomycin/polymyxin B) alone or in combination with a topical corticosteroid.

The combination of a topical antibiotic and a corticosteroid such as betamethasone is safe and effective for the treatment of uncomplicated acute bacterial paronychia and seems to offer advantages compared with topical antibiotics alone.

For persistent lesions, oral antistaphylococcal antibiotic therapy should be used in conjunction with warm soaks. Patients with exposure to oral flora via finger sucking or hangnail biting should be treated against anaerobes with a broad-spectrum oral antibiotic (e.g., amoxicillin/clavulanate, clindamycin) because of possible *S. aureus* and Bacteroides resistance to penicillin and ampicillin. If there is concern for methicillin resistant *S. aureus*, clindamycin or trimethoprim-sulfamethoxazole are considered good choices for therapy. Alternative options include doxycycline, minocycline, and linezolid.

> Avoid trimming cuticles or using cuticle removers.

Surgical treatment

Surgical intervention for paronychia is generally recommended when an abscess is present. Antibiotics are generally not needed after successful drainage. Prospective studies have shown that the addition of systemic antibiotics does not improve cure rates after incision and drainage of cutaneous abscesses, even in those due to methicillin-resistant *S. aureus*. Post-drainage soaking with or without Burow's solution or 1% acetic acid is generally recommended twice or three times per day for two to three days.

Superficial infections can be easily drained with a size-11 scalpel or a comedone extractor. Pain is quickly relieved after drainage. Another simple technique to drain a paronychial abscess involves lifting the nail fold with the tip of a 21- or 23-gauge needle, followed immediately by passive oozing of pus from the nail bed; this technique does not require anesthesia or daily dressing. If there is no clear response within 2 days, deep surgical incision under local anesthesia (digital proximal nerve block) may be needed, particularly in children. The proximal one-third of the nail plate can be removed without initial incisional drainage. This technique gives more rapid relief and more sustained drainage, especially in patients with paronychia resulting from an ingrown nail. Complicated infections can occur in immunosuppressed patients and in patients with diabetes or untreated infections.

Surgical treatment of chronic paronychia

If protective measures and corticosteroids (topical or intralesional), or tacrolimus and topical antimicrobials or antifungals are ineffective, surgery is mandatory.

Marsupialization is no longer in use. We prefer the technique we have described: a crescent-shaped full thickness of the proximal nail fold. We excise a full-thickness piece of the proximal nail fold, that is 4–5 mm at its greatest width, and extends from one lateral nail fold to the other and includes more or less the entire swollen portion of the fold. Complete healing by secondary intention takes about one month.

In patients who experience repeated acute painful flares associated with chronic paronychia, removal of the base of the nail plate is useful, total nail avulsion being rarely necessary.

The latest surgical technique decribed by a Brazilian team removes only the ventral fibrotic tissue of the proximal and lateral nail folds. This elegant technique minimizes nail fold retraction and recovery time with optimal cosmetic results.

> - Avoid nail trauma, biting, picking, manipulation, and finger sucking.
> - Keep affected areas clean and dry.
> - Provide adequate patient education.
> - Improve glycemic control in patients with diabetes.

FURTHER READING

Baran R., Bureau H. (1991) Surgical treatment of recalcitrant chronic paronychia. *J. Dermatol Surg Oncol*; 7: 106–107.

Ferreira Vieira d'Almeida L., Papaiordanou F., Araujo Machado E. et al. (2016) Chronic paronychia treatment: square flap technique. *JAAD*; 75: 398-03.

Kirkland E. B., Adams B. B. (2008) Methicillin-resistant *Staphylococcus aureus* and athletes. *J Am Acad Dermatol*; 59(3): 494–502.

Leggit J. C. (2017 Jul 1) Acute and chronic paronychia. *Am Fam Physician*; 96(1): 44–51.

Rigopoulos D., Larios G., Gregoriou S., et al. (2008) Acute and chronic paronychia. *AmFam Physician*; 77: 339–346.

Rigopoulos D., Gregoriou S., Belyayeva Y., et al. (2009) Acute paronychia caused by lapatinib therapy. *Clin Exp Dermatol*; 34: 94–95.

Sezer E., Bridges A. G., Koseoglu D., et al. (2009) Acquired periungual fibrokeratoma developing after acute Staphylococcal paronychia. *Eur J Dermatol*; 19: 636–637.

11

Chronic paronychia

Dimitris Rigopoulos

Chronic paronychia is a multifactorial inflammatory reaction of the proximal nail fold to irritants and allergens. Women are affected more frequently than men, and the condition is usually seen on the hands.

This disorder can be the result of numerous conditions such as dishwashing, finger sucking, aggressively trimming the cuticles, and frequent contact with chemicals (e.g., mild alkalis, acids) Allergens and irritants comprise the major pathogenetic factors, as suggested by the increased prevalence of the disorder among laundry workers, house and office cleaners, food handlers, cooks, dishwashers, bartenders, chefs, fishmongers, and nurses. Sensitization to allergens as suggested by patch testing is also high in patients with chronic paronychia. In chronic paronychia, the cuticle separates from the nail plate, leaving the region between the proximal nail fold and the nail plate vulnerable to infection by bacterial and fungal pathogens (Figure 11.1).

There is some disagreement over the importance and role of Candida in chronic paronychia. *Candida* sp. is often isolated in patients with chronic paronychia. Several studies using topical or systemic antifungals in the treatment of chronic paronychia have reported encouraging results. However, investigators have suggested that the therapeutic potential of antifungals in chronic paronychia might be attributed equally to the antifungal and to the anti-inflammatory properties of the agents. Even in studies showing a good therapeutic effect, some of the patients reported unsuccessful antifungal therapy in the past. In addition, it has been shown that 50% of the patients in these studies present an immediate type hypersensitivity to Candida antigens in intradermal tests, which is not shared by controls. The relation of this finding to the pathogenesis and duration of chronic paronychia has not been clarified adequately. Tosti and others (2002) demonstrated that the presence of Candida is not linked to disease activity and established the superiority of topical steroids over antifungal agents in the treatment of chronic paronychia.

Chronic paronychia can result as a complication of acute paronychia in patients who do not receive appropriate treatment. Chronic paronychia often occurs in people with diabetes.

The use of systemic drugs, such as retinoids and protease inhibitors (e.g., indinavir and lamivudine), may cause chronic paronychia.

Indinavir is the most common cause of chronic or recurrent paronychia of the toes or fingers in people infected with a human immunodeficiency virus. The mechanism of indinavir-induced retinoid-like effects is unclear. Paronychia has also been reported in patients taking cetuximab, an anti-epidermal growth factor receptor (EGFR) antibody used in the treatment of solid tumors. Chronic paronychia can also present as possible adverse event associated with systemic drugs, such as taxanes, EGFR inhibitors, EGFR tyrosine kinase inhibitors, BRAF inhibitors, CD20 antagonists, vascular endothelial growth factor inhibitors, and retinoids.

- One or several fingernails are usually affected and typically the thumb and second or third finger of the dominant hand.
- Avoid or treat predisposing conditions. Educate the patient as to proper nail care.
- The nail plate becomes thickened and discolored, with pronounced transverse ridges such as Beau's lines (resulting from inflammation of the nail matrix) and nail loss.

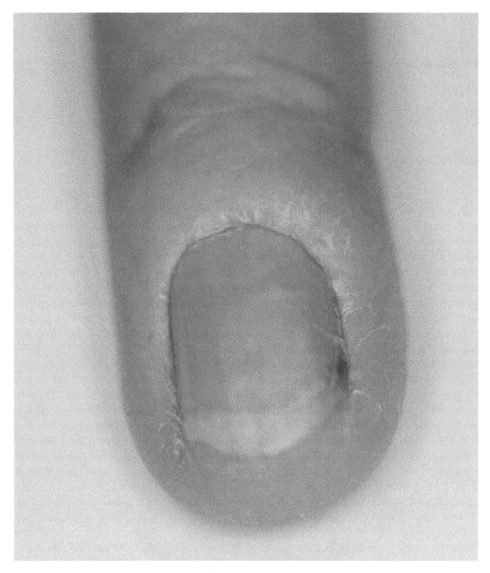

FIGURE 11.1 Chronic paronychia with slight fissures of the proximal nail fold associated with desquamating tissue.

TABLE 11.1

Signs of Chronic Paronychia

Erythema

Tenderness on pressure of the PNF

Swelling of the nail fold

Absence of the adjacent cuticle

Pus may form below the nail fold

Blackish lateral edges with fine transverse grooves

Note: PNF, proximal nail fold.

Grading

- Stage I: Redness, some swelling of the cuticle/proximal nail fold that may or may not cause disruption of the cuticle seal.
- Stage II: Redness and pronounced swelling of the proximal nail fold and disruption of the cuticle seal.
- Stage III: Redness and swelling of the proximal nail fold, absent cuticle, some discomfort, early edema, some nail plate changes.
- Stage IV: Redness and swelling of the proximal nail fold, absent cuticle, tender/painful, edema, extensive nail plate changes.
- Stage V: Same as stage IV plus acute exacerbation of chronic paronychia (acute paronychia).

A new severity index for the evaluation of chronic paronychia has been proposed by Atis (2019), based on the involvement of the nail folds, on the presence of erythema, oedema, on changes of the cuticle and the nail plate.

Treatment

Patients should wear cotton and vinyl gloves when peeling or squeezing citrus fruits, handling tomatoes, and peeling potatoes or other raw food. They should also avoid direct contact with paint, metal polish, paint thinner, solvents, and polish and wear cotton and vinyl gloves when using them. They should use lukewarm water and very mild soap when washing hands, be sure to rinse the soap off and dry hands gently.

Leave the cuticle alone! Do not cut it. Do not push it back with another fingernail, metal file, or stick.

A broad-spectrum topical antifungal agent can be used to treat the condition and prevent recurrence (amorolfine has given interesting results in some cases).

Application of emollient lotions to lubricate the nascent cuticle and the hands is usually beneficial. One randomized controlled trial assigned 45 adults with chronic paronychia to treatment with a systemic antifungal agent (itraconazole or terbinafine) or a topical steroid cream (methylprednisolone aceponate) for 3 weeks. After 9 weeks, more patients in the topical steroid group were improved or cured (91 vs 49%; $P < 0.01$; number needed to treat = 2.4).

The presence or absence of Candida seems to be unrelated to the effectiveness of treatment.

Given their lower risks and costs compared with systemic antifungals, topical steroids should be the first-line treatment for patients with chronic paronychia. Alternatively, topical treatment with a combination of steroid and antifungal agents may also be used in patients with simple chronic paronychia, although data showing the superiority of this treatment to steroid use alone are lacking.

Paronychia induced by the EGFR inhibitor cetuximab can be treated with an antibiotic such as doxycycline. In patients with paronychia induced by indinavir, substitution of an alternative anti-retroviral regimen that retains lamivudine and other protease inhibitors can resolve retinoid-like manifestations without recurrences.

In an unblinded randomized study, the efficacy of tacrolimus ointment 0.1% was compared with that of betamethasone 17-valerate 0.1% or placebo, in the treatment of chronic paronychia. Tacrolimus ointment appears to be a more efficacious agent, for the treatment of chronic paronychia than betamethasone or a placebo.

A case report describes successful treatment with twice-daily application of a 1% solution of povi-done/iodine in dimethyl sulfoxide until symptom resolution in patients with chemotherapy-induced chronic paronychia.

Intralesional corticosteroid administration (triamcinolone) may be used in refractory cases. Systemic corticosteroids may be used for the treatment of inflammation and pain for a limited period in patients with severe paronychia involving several fingernails.

If patients with chronic paronychia do not respond to topical therapy and avoidance of contact with water and irritants, a trial of systemic antifungals may be useful before attempting invasive approaches. Further, treatment with 20 mg of supplemental zinc per day is helpful in cases of zinc deficiency.

Surgical Treatment/Lasers

In patients with recalcitrant chronic paronychia, en bloc excision of 4–5 mm of the proximal nail fold (PNF) is effective. Simultaneous avulsion of the nail plate (total or partial, restricted to the base of the nail plate and lateral edges) improves the surgical outcome. Alternatively, crescentic excision may be performed. This technique involves excision of a semi-circular skin section proximal to the nail fold and parallel to the eponychium, expanding to the edge of the nail fold on both sides (the vertical part of the PNF remains exposed and it can be infected).

A pilot study was conducted to assess the role of 1064 Nd:YAG laser for the treatment of chronic paronychia. The results demonstrated that seven of eight patients showed an apparent clinical improvement without side effects, and therefore Nd:YAG laser therapy seems to be an alternate promising and safe method.

- Chronic paronychia has been present for at least 6 weeks at the time of diagnosis.
- The condition usually has a prolonged course with recurrent, self-limited episodes of acute exacerbation.
- Wear light cotton gloves under heavy-duty vinyl gloves for wet work.
- Chronic paronychia responds slowly to treatment. Resolution usually takes several weeks or months, but the slow improvement rate should not discourage physicians and patients.
- In mild to moderate cases, 9 weeks of drug treatment is usually effective.
- Patients with chronic toenail paronychia that is unresponsive to standard treatment should be investigated for unusual causes, such as malignancy.

BIBLIOGRAPHY

Atış G. Göktay F. AltanFerhatoğlu Z, et al. (2018 Nov) A proposal for a New Severity Index for the Evaluation of Chronic Paronychia. *Skin Appendage Disord*; 5(1), 32–33.

Capriotti K. Capriotti J. A. (2015) Chemotherapy-associated paronychia treated with a dilute povidone-iodine/dimethylsulfoxide preparation. *Clin Cosmet Investig Dermatol*; 8, 489–491.

El-Komy M. H. Samir N (2015 Jul) 1064 Nd:YAG laser for the treatment of chronic paronychia: a pilot study. *Lasers Med Sci*; 30(5), 1623–1626.

Iorizzo M. (2015) Tips to treat the 5 most common nail disorders: brittle nails, onycholysis, paronychia, psoriasis, onychomycosis. *Dermatol Clin*; 33(2), 175–183.

Lomax A. Thornton J. Singh D. (2016 Dec) Toenail paronychia. *Foot Ankle Surg*; 22(4), 219–223.

Rao A. Bunker C (2010) Efficacy and safety of tacrolimus ointment 0.1% vs. betamethasone 17-valerate 0.1% in the treatment of chronic paronychia: an unblinded randomized study. *Br J Dermatol*; 163, 208.

Rigopoulos D. Larios G. Gregoriou S, et al. (2008) Acute and chronic paronychia. *Am Fam Physician*; 77: 339–346.

Rigopoulos D. Gregoriou S. Belyayeva E., et al. (2009) Efficacy and safety of tacrolimus ointment 0.1% vs. betamethasone 17-valerate 0.1% in the treatment of chronic paronychia: an unblinded randomized study. *Br J Dermatol*; 160, 858–860.

Tosti A. Piraccini B. M., Ghetti E., et al. (2002) Topical steroids versus systemic antifungals in the treatment of chronic paronychia: an open, randomized double-blind and double dummy study. *J Am Acad Dermatol*; 47, 73–76.

Wollina U. (2018 Sep–Oct) Systemic drug-induced chronic paronychia and periungual pyogenic granuloma. *Indian Dermatol Online J*; 9(5), 293–298.

12

Warts

Dimitris Rigopoulos

Pathogen

Human papillomaviruses (HPV) constitute a heterogeneous group of more than 100 different types of viruses distinguished by DNA sequence analysis. DNA virus 1, 2, 4 cause most periungual warts, and HPV 7 causes butchers' warts. HPV associated with skin lesions are classified as cutaneous HPV, which are different from the genital HPV. The difference between cutaneous types and genital types of HPV is that the cutaneous types do not have the E5 open reading frame (except for a few cutaneous types) compared with the genital types.

Periungual warts are most frequently encountered in teenagers between 12 and 16 years (Figure 12.1). They are usually found in the proximal and lateral nail folds, as well as in the hyponychium and from there they can invade the nail bed but not directly the nail matrix. Despite this fact, warts can affect the nail matrix, producing nail plate ridging and grooving. The penetration of the virus is favored by skin abrasion and maceration. These facts explain why periungual warts are commonly found in nail biters, children who suck their fingers, and people working in a wet environment. In some cases, warts of the proximal nail fold can appear with significant edema of the proximal nail fold, resembling a reaction to a foreign body (Figure 12.2).

Patients with periungual warts who bite their fingers should be examined for warts on their lips and face.

The inoculation time of warts is from a few weeks up to 1 year.

Periungual warts are usually asymptomatic, and pain can result from fissuring of the warts or due to their subungual growth.

Both humoral and cellular immunity are important in the host response to the HPV infection, so immunodeficiency, both primary and secondary, are associated with persistent wart infection.

Subungual warts have rarely been described to be associated with bone erosions. X-ray when needed.

TABLE 12.1

Signs of Warts

Rough surface
Hyperkeratotic
Papillomatous
Skin-colored

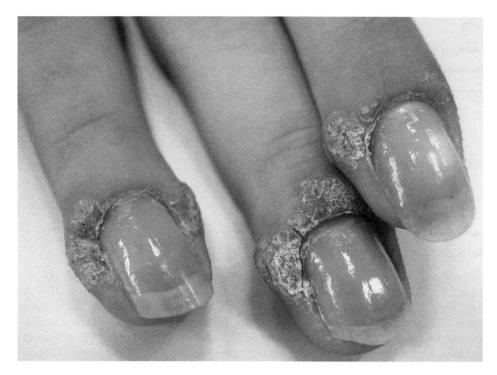

FIGURE 12.1   Periungual warts.

Diagnosis

Diagnosis is usually easy and is based on the clinical appearance. Sometimes, especially when they are situated subungually, biopsy with PCR detection of the virus or Southern blot hybridization may be needed in order to specify the type of the infection responsible for the HPV virus.

Transillumination, the technique of sample illumination by transmission of light through the sample, can be used as a simple tool to assess the subungual extent of periungual warts.

HPV cannot be cultured.

Prognosis

About (25%) of the warts may disappear within 6 months and 65% within 2 years.

Treatment

There is no single method of treatment that is universally effective. Treatment should be tailored to each individual patient need.

Periungual and subungual warts are difficult to treat, but aggressive treatment modalities are unnecessary, especially in children.

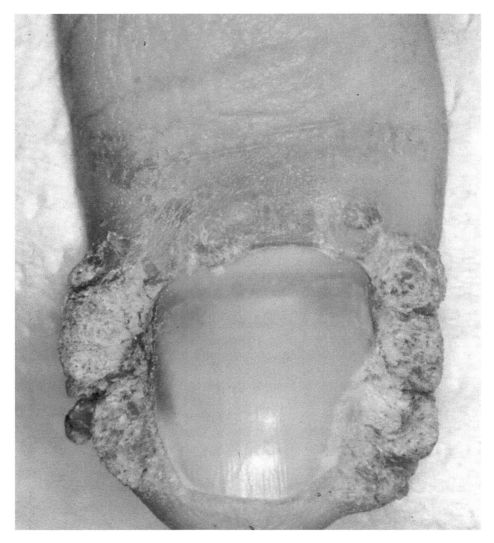

FIGURE 12.2 Periungual warts resembling foreign body reaction.

The number of warts, exact location, age of the patient, and the doctor's experience are some of the factors that influence, which treatment the expert will choose.

Long-standing periungual warts should alert the expert to the development of Bowen's disease or squamous cell carcinoma. In most cases, HPV 16 is detected.

Topical Treatments

1. Peeling agents
2. Cantharidin
3. Imiquimod

4. Immunotherapy
5. Virucidal agents
6. Nitric oxide releasing solutions
7. Formic acid
8. Alternative treatments

1. **Peeling or keratolytic agents** are extremely popular for the treatment of children presenting with warts. These contain salicylic acid alone in a concentration of 10%–40% or in combination with lactic acid. They are usually found in the form of creams, ointments, tapes, or quick-drying acrylate lacquers. For best results and increased penetration, the affected area can be hydrated by soaking in warm water for 5–10 minutes, before application of any of these agents.
2. **Cantharidin** 19% with salicylic acid 30% and podophyllin 2% in flexible collodion can be applied in a thin coat for 4–6 hours under occlusion, with excellent results.
3. **Imiquimod** is a local inducer of cytokine, especially interferon-alpha. It is used in the form of a 5% cream, at bedtime and should be kept topically for 6–10 hours and then washed off. Topical imiquimod achieves a complete resolution of 80% of subungual and periungual warts, after a mean time of 3 weeks. This is an "off-label" use, as it is approved for genital warts, actinic keratosis, and BCC.
4. **Immunotherapy** with topical squaric acid dibutylether or diphenylcyclopropenone used once a week is effective in the treatment of resistant warts. They act as strong topical sensitizers. Of the patients using this method, 87.7% achieved clearance with an average of five treatments over a 6-month period.

   Injections of vitamin D3 solution can be given at a dose of $0.1\ mL/cm^2$ just beneath the wart. A maximum of 0.4 mL is used in a single session in cases with multiple warts. The session can be repeated at 2-week intervals for a maximum of 4 sessions or until complete resolution of warts, whichever is earlier. It is a safe, inexpensive, effective management option for periungual warts.

   Immunotherapy with 0.1 ml of killed Mycobacterium w vaccine, given intralesionally at four weekly intervals, has also shown high cure rates.
5. **Glutaraldehyde** and formaldehyde can have therapeutic effect comparable to that of keratolytic agents.
6. **Nitric–zinc complex solution (NZCS)** is a topically applied solution containing nitric acid, zinc, copper, and organic acids that induce a painless caustic effect on "difficult-to-treat" warts, including periungual locations. In a study with a pediatric population with palmoplantar and periungual warts, NZCS resulted in complete wart clearance in 83.9% and had excellent cosmetic effects. This approach is easy to use, with extremely low discomfort levels, and represents a good treatment option particularly in this special population.
7. Topical puncture with **formic acid** 85% solution has been used in a series of 34 patients, with good results. In France, this is sold as an over-the-counter substance for adults and children over 4 years old, for once-a-week topical use.
8. A large part of therapy is the psychological component.

According to the geographical region, many alternative treatment modalities are used, especially on children. The use of an ordinary roll of tape, but labeled "WART TAPE" is used by some dermatologists. The tape is wrapped around the finger with much ceremony and kept on for 6 days and replaced the following morning. According to the author of the article, 80% cure rate was seen after 4 weeks.

Another alternative way of treating periungual warts is to immerse the affected finger in 45° water for 30 minutes, three times a week.

As mentioned previously, periungual warts are a common complication in nail biters and the use of a distasteful preparation such as 4% quinine in petrolatum, quaternary amino derivates on the dorsum of the distal phalanges may be useful. In women, a habit-tic may be discouraged by a regimen of nail care, particularly through the use of color or nail art helping the patient to protect their nails from injury.

Systemic Treatments

1. Immunomodulators
2. Interferons
3. antimitotic agents

1. Cimetidine is an H2 receptor antagonist that has proven to be an immunomodulator, probably blocking H2 receptors from suppressing T cells, increasing cell immunity. Administration of cimetidine increases proliferation of lymphocytes, inhibits the function of suppressing T cells and enhances the reactivity of skin tests. It has been successfully used to stimulate the immune system of patients with T cell immunodeficiency. Cimetidine has been used in the treatment of urticaria, mastocytosis, different eosinophilic dermatoses, warts, external condyloma acuminatum, molluscum contagiosum, and epidermodysplasia verruciformis. The incidence of adverse reactions is low and normally minimum, below 3%. Use of high dose cimetidine, 30–40 mg/kg, in the treatment of viral warts has been reported in literature in recent years, but with conflicting results. However, current data do not support the use of H2-antagonists for the treatment of common warts.

   A meta-analysis study performed by Salman and others (2019) showed the efficacy of intralesional immunotherapeutic modalities, especially PPD and MMR, favoring over some destructive modalities, such as cryotherapy. In contrast to PPD, the MMR vaccine is not recommended during pregnancy.

2. One patient with recalcitrant subungual and periungual warts was treated with intravenous human fibroblast beta interferon (3 cycles, 14 days each; daily dose $1–3 \times 10^6$ IU). Complete remission of all warts was achieved. One year after treatment, the patient was still free of any wart.

3. A solution of bleomycin (a cytotoxic polypeptide, which acts by binding to the viral DNA in warts and prevents replication, leading to cell death) (1U bleomycin X 1 ml sterile saline), after topical anesthesia with EMLA (lidocaine and prilocaine 1:1), is dropped on to the wart and "pricked" into the wart using a needle, for approximately 40 times per 5 mm^2. The wart is slowly necrotized with the formation of an eschar after 3–4 weeks of treatment, which then can be removed. Intralesional bleomycin is a rather painful procedure; clinicians do not choose it for the treatment of periungual or subungual warts, except as bleopuncture under local anesthesia (without epinephrine) followed by nail removal in subungual location. In a recent study, the intralesional use of bleomycin associated with electroporation for the treatment of ungual warts showed a statistically superior cure when compared with intralesional bleomycin alone.

Surgical Treatments

- When using cryotherapy do not overfreeze as the underlying nail matrix can be affected and produce leukonychia or onychomadesis and in some cases, atrophy of the nail plate.
- In the case of periungual hyperkeratotic warts, these should be pared off before freezing in order to permit deeper tissue freezing.
- Best treatment for warts at the hyponychium and at the nail folds is bleopuncture.

1. Cryotherapy
2. Laser treatment
   - CO_2
   - Pulsed dye laser
   - Er:YAG

3. Photodynamic therapy (PDT)

4. Electrocautery

5. Surgery

1. Cryotherapy with liquid nitrogen (−196°C to −320.8°F) can be applied with a cotton swab or with a cryotherapy gun. An aerosol spray with adapter freeze at −70°C (−94°F) is also available as an OTC in some countries and self-used by the patients with variable results. It is not considered as first-line treatment for young children, as it is rather painful.

    In the case of periungual hyperkeratotic warts, the hyperkeratosis should be pared off before freezing, in order to permit deeper tissue freezing. Time of freezing ranges between 10 and 15 seconds.

    The wart is frozen until 1–2 mm of surrounding skin has turned white. Generally, the cure rates approach 90%.

    Onychomadesis, leukonychia, and Beau's lines can develop on the nail plate, due to damage of the underlying nail matrix (in the case of warts situated on the proximal nail fold). Nail atrophy, which can be permanent, is rather infrequent, but can happen

2. Laser treatment
    - CO_2 laser: Vaporization of the tissue of periungual warts with CO_2 laser seems to be effective in the majority of cases. Pain can occur, but in most cases, it is short lived and manageable. One or two sessions are usually needed. The most important short-coming and side effects of CO_2 laser are the prolonged healing and postoperative process and the high cost of the instrument. Infections and significant onychodystrophy are uncommon.
    - Pulse dye laser 585 and 595 nm: The principal action of this type of laser is the destruction of the capillaries of the wart, as these wavelengths are absorbed by oxyhemoglobin. Cure rates of periungual warts after 2–4 sessions do not exceed 35% of the cases.
    - Er:YAG laser: This type of laser produces a controlled tissue ablation, with minimal thermal damage compared with the CO_2 laser. Langdon has used this type of laser with an excellent safety profile, minimal morbidity, minimal pain, and no injected anesthesia.

3. Photodynamic therapy: This is a new treatment modality for periungual warts, which entails the administration of an exogenous photosensitizer (in this case, 20% d-aminolevulinic acid-ALA in the form of a cream, which is applied 3–6 hours prior to radiation). It is preferentially taken up by malignant and abnormal cells and transformed into photosensitizing porphyrin. The photodynamic effect involves the excitation of the photosensitizer by light of the appropriate wavelength (in this case 580–720 nm was used, which was applied with a fluence of 100 nW/CM2 for 5–30 min), resulting in the formation of toxic radicals, which are directly destructive to the tissues. The mechanism of action of PDT involves both a direct killing of the tumor cells and a secondary effect resulting from vascular damage. A 100% clearance rate in 90% of the patients was achieved with this method. The average number of treatments was 4–5. This is a noninvasive method without any scars or nail deformities. Pain is minimal, so it is suitable for young children. Duration of the treatment is a disadvantage, as is the number of treatments needed.

4. Electrocautery: This method should not be used to treat periungual warts, as it results in scarring.

5. Surgery: Poor wound healing, trauma, painful scarring, bleeding, and prolonged discomfort have caused this method to fall out of favor.

BIBLIOGRAPHY

AlGhamdi K. M., Khurram H. (2011) Successful treatment of periungual warts with diluted bleomycin using translesional multipuncture technique: a pilot prospective study. *DermatolSurg*; 37: 486–492.

Ashique K. T., Kaliyadan F. (2013 Apr-Jun) Transillumination: a simple tool to assess subungual extension in periungual warts. *Indian Dermatol Online J*; 4(2): 131–132.

Chern E., Cheng Y. W. (2010) Treatment of recalcitrant periungual warts with cimetidine in pediatrics. *J Dermatolog Treat*; 21: 314–316.

Di Chiacchio N. G., Di Chiacchio N., Criado P. R., Brunner C. H. M., Suaréz M. V. R., Belda Junior W. (2019 Dec) Ungual warts: comparison of treatment with intralesional bleomycin and electroporation in terms of efficacy and safety. *JEADV*; 33(12): 2349–2354.

Faghihi G., Vali A., Radan M., et al. (2010 Mar-Apr) A double-blind, randomized trial of local formic acid puncture technique in the treatment of common warts. *Skinmed*; 8(2): 70–71.

Garg S., Baveja S. (2014 Oct–Dec) Intralesional immunotherapy for difficult to treat warts with Mycobacterium w vaccine. *J Cutan Aesthet Surg*; 7(4): 203–208.

Giacaman A., Granger C., Aladren S., Bauzá A., Alomar Torrens B., Riutort Mercant M., Martin-Santiago A. (2019 Dec) Use of topical nitric–zinc complex solution to treat palmoplantar and periungual warts in a pediatric population. *Dermatol Ther (Heidelb)*; 9(4): 755–760.

Jakhar D., Kaur I., Misri R. (2019 May) Intralesional vitamin D3 in periungual warts. *J Am Acad Dermatol*; 80(5): e111–e112.

Matsukura T., Sugase M. (2001) Relationships between 80 human papillomavirus genotypes and different grades of cervical intraepithelial neoplasia: association and causality. *Virology*; 283: 139.

Micali G., Dall'Oglio F., Nasca M. R. (2003) An open label evaluation of the efficacy of imiquimod 5% cream in the treatment of recalcitrant subungual and periungual cutaneous warts. *J Dermatol Treat*; 14: 233–236.

Moore A. Y. (2009) Clinical applications for topical 5-fluorouracil in the treatment of dermatological disorders. *J Dermatol Treat*; 20: 328–335.

Rampen F. H., Steijlen P. M. (1996) Diphencyprone in the management of refractory palmoplantar and periungual warts: an open study. *Dermatology*; 193: 236–238.

Salman S., Ahmed M. S., Ibrahim A. M., et al. (2019 Apr) Intralesional immunotherapy for the treatment of warts: A network meta-analysis. *JAAD*; 80(4): 922–930.

Sardana K., Garg V., Relhan V. (2010) Complete resolution of recalcitrant periungual/subungual wart with recovery of normal nail following "prick" method of administration of bleomycin 1%. *Dermatol Ther*; 23: 407–410.

Tosti A., Piraccini B. M. (2001 Mar) Warts of the nail unit: surgical and nonsurgical approaches. *Dermatol Surg*; 27(3): 235–239.

13

Yellow nail syndrome

Dimitris Rigopoulos
Robert Baran

Yellow nail syndrome (YNS), first described in 1964, is an uncommon disorder which is characterized by the presence of yellow nails (Figure 13.1), lymphedema, and diverse respiratory manifestations, such as pleural effusion, bronchiectasis, rhinosinusitis, chronic cough, or recurrent lung infections. It has been reported that congenital malformations and a secondary dysfunction of lymphatic vessels may be responsible for the syndrome, but the exact mechanism is still not known. More recently, microvasculopathy with protein leakage has been suggested as a more likely culprit.

The time between the developments of the various manifestations of the syndrome may range from months to years.

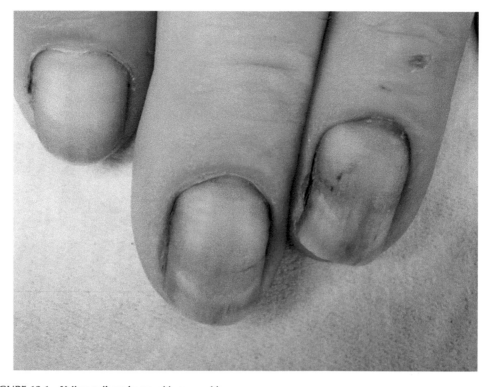

FIGURE 13.1   Yellow nail syndrome with paronychia.

Some authors have classified YNS as a hereditary disorder, transmitted in an autosomal dominant fashion, while others have linked YNS to a variety of underlying diseases, including connective tissue disease, malignancy, immunodeficiency states, endocrine disorders including diabetes mellitus and thyroid dysfunction, or as an adverse drug effect (e.g., penicillamine, bucillamine, or gold sodium thiomalate). All three criteria may not be simultaneously present, and two of them have been judged to be sufficient for diagnosis. The complete triad is seen in only 30%–60% of cases. YNS is usually found between the fourth and sixth decades of life, while it is rarely seen in children. Stemmer's sign (inability to pinch the skin on the dorsal side on the base of the 2nd toe), which yields a definitive lymphedema diagnosis, is positive in these patients (Table 13.1).

Rule out nail fungal or *Pseudomonas* infection.

Various investigations to establish the diagnosis may be conducted (Table 13.2).

TABLE 13.1

Signs of Yellow Nail Syndrome

Slow nail growth (less than 0.2 mm/week)
Marked thickening
Yellow to yellow-green discoloration
Excessively curved nail plate
Absent lunula
Swelling of the periungual tissue
Onycholysis
Hardness of the nail plate
Chronic paronychia (occasionally)

TABLE 13.2

Possible Investigations for Yellow Nail Syndrome

Complete blood count
Urinalysis and evaluation of proteinuria
Immuno-electrophoresis
Thyroid-stimulating hormone
Waaler-Rose test for serum rheumatoid factors
Chemistry profile with blood creatinine
Sinus and chest radiography
Cone beam computed tomography
Ear, nose, and throat and pulmonary investigations
Liver enzymes, alkaline phosphatases
Exposure to Titanium Dioxide
• Foods such as candy, chewing gum and chocolate
• Personal care items, such as shampoo, sunscreen, and toothpaste
• Drugs such as multivitamins

Treatment

YNS treatment options are limited and often unsuccessful.

Patients can conceal their nails with nail enamel, although this may not be always possible.

Spontaneous resolution of the nail changes has been reported. Intradermal injections of triamcinolone in the proximal nail fold have been reported to be useful. Vitamin E in high doses of 500I U twice a day, probably due to the antioxidant properties of alpha tocopherol, can induce complete resolution of the nail changes. Tocopherol has also been used with pulses of fluconazole, 300 mg once weekly, which is well known for increasing the rate of linear growth of the nail. This drug combination has been reported as giving very promising results.

Of course, treatment of any concomitant disease is mandatory.

Topical vitamin E solution in dimethyl sulfoxide has been shown to be effective in the treatment of nail changes in YNS.

Oral zinc supplementation for 2 years, dietary restriction of fat, and supplements of medium-chain triglycerides and octreotide, which is a somatostatin (growth hormone-inhibiting hormone) analog, were reported to be successful in dealing with nail changes in the syndrome.

- Complete triad of the syndrome is seen in approximately 30%–60% of cases.
- α-Tocopherol and azoles are considered as first-line treatment for YNS.
- Treatment of associated malignancy, if any, may improve the syndrome.

FURTHER READING

Al Hawsawi K., Pope E. (2010) Yellow nail syndrome. *Pediatr Dermatol*; 27, 675–676.

Avitan-Hersh E., Berger G., Bergman R. (2011) Yellow nail syndrome. *Isr Med Assoc J*; 13, 577–578.

Baran R., Thomas L. (2009) Combination of fluconazole and alpha-tocopherol in the treatment of yellow nail syndrome. *J Drugs Dermatol*; 8, 276–278.

Cordasco E. M. Jr, Beder S., Coltro A., et al. (1990) Clinical features of the yellow nail syndrome. *Cleve Clin J Med*; 57, 472–476.

Dos Santos V. M. (2016) Titanium pigment and yellow nail syndrome. *Skin Appendage Disorders*; 1(4):197.

Hillerdal G. (2007) Yellow nail syndrome: treatment with octreotide. *Clin Respir J*; 1, 120–121.

Hoque S. R., Mansour S., Mortimer P. S. (2007) Yellow nail syndrome: not a genetic disorder? Eleven new cases and a review of the literature. *Br J Dermatol*; 156, 1230–1234.

Iheonunekwu N., Adedayo O., Clare A., Cummings C. (2011) Yellow nail syndrome in a medical clinic. *West Indian Med J*; 60, 99–101.

Vignes S., Baran R. (2017 Feb 27) Yellow nail syndrome: a review. *Orphanet J Rare Dis*; 12(1), 42.

14

Onycholysis

Robert Baran

Onycholysis is a common disorder with nail plate-nail bed separation leading to a whitish appearance due to the nail transparency (Figure 14.1). The pattern of separation of the plate from the nail bed takes many forms. Sometimes, it closely resembles the damage from a splinter under the nail that is the detachment extending proximally along a convex line, giving the appearance of a half-moon. When the process reaches the matrix, onycholysis becomes complete. Involvement of the lateral edge of the nail alone is less common; in certain cases, the free edge rises up like a hood, or coils open itself like a

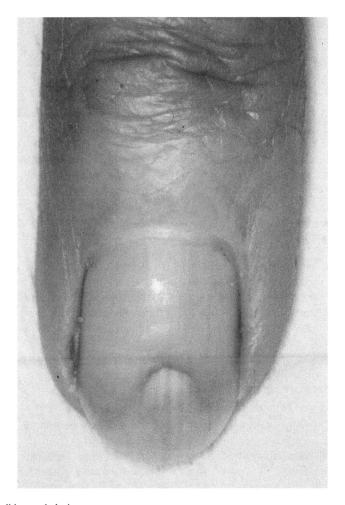

FIGURE 14.1 Candida onycholysis.

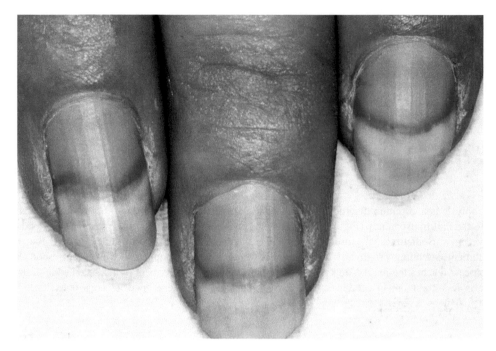

FIGURE 14.2 Nail psoriasis with its proximal red margin.

roll of paper. Onycholysis creates a subungual space that gathers dirt and keratin debris. After a more or less period of onycholysis, the nail bed may epithelialize, leading to a phenomenon that has been sometimes named "disappearing" nail bed (Daniel, Tosti, Iorizzo, and Piraccini 2017) different from that observed with local corticoids, especially in children (see chapter). The grayish-white color, sometimes observed, is due to the presence of air under the nail, but the color may vary from yellow to green or brown, depending on the etiology. In psoriasis, there is usually a red margin visible between the normal pink nail and the separate white onycholytic area (Figure 14.2).

Primary onycholysis may be associated with the presence of Candida in fingernail. Mixed infection due to *Candida* and *Pseudomonas* is not rare and is sometimes malodorous. Onycholysis associated with oozing should bring to mind Bowen's disease and transillumination of the terminal phalanx gives a good view of this area.

The onset of this condition may be sudden, due to drugs (Table 14.1), as in photo-onycholysis (Table 14.2) with its triad of photosensitization, onycholysis, and dyschromia (Figure 14.3). Occupation (Table 14.3) may be the cause when there is a contact with chemical irritants, such as hydrofluoric acid or thioglycolate. Sculptured onycholysis is a self-induced nail abnormality produced by cleaning the underside of the nail plate with a sharp instrument. In fact, onycholysis may be associated with various conditions (Table 14.4).

Onycholysis of the toes demonstrates some differences from that of the fingers:

- Lack of occupational hazards
- Reduced use of cosmetics on the toes
- Protection afforded by footwear which reduces the risk of onycholysis

The two main causes of onycholysis of the toes are onychomycosis primarily due to *Trichophyton rubrum* and "trauma exerted by the closed shoes on the toes because of an "Asymmetric gait due to ubiquitous and even flat feet," sometimes called *AGnus* (Zaias, Escovar, and Zaias 2015).

TABLE 14.1

Drugs That Can Cause Onycholysis

5-fluorouracil	Fluoroquinolones
Adriamycin	Minocycline
Aripiprazole	Mitoxantrone
Benoxaprofen	Olanzapine
Bleomycin	Oral contraceptives
Capecitabine	Paclitaxel
Chloramphenicol	Photodynamic treatment
Chlorpromazine	Psoralens
Chlortetracycline	Retinoids
Cytotoxic	Roxithromycin
Dimethylchlortetracycline	Tetracycline and its derivatives
Doxycycline	

TABLE 14.2

Drug-Induced Photo-Onycholysis

Antibiotics	Tetracyclines (especially demethylchlortetracycline, doxycycline, less frequently minocyclines, tetracycline hydrochloride, oxytetracycline, chlortetracycline)
	Cephaloridine, cloxacillin, chloramphenicol (uncommon)
	Fluoroquinolones (sparfloxacin), moxifloxacin
	Cephaloridine, cloxacillin, chloramphenicol (uncommon)
Antipsychotics	Olanzapine, aripiprazole
Psoralens with sunlight or UVA	8-methoxypsoralen
	5-methoxypsoralen
	Trimethylpsoralen
Appropriate light source for PDT	Photodynamic onycholysis (methyl aminolevulinate)
Miscellaneous	Acriflavine
	Benoxaprofen
	Captopril
	Chlorazepate dipotassium
	Chlorpromazine
	Icodextrine
	Indapamide
	Indomethacin
	Oral contraceptives
	Paroxetine
	Quinine
	Sirolimus
	Thiazide diuretics
	Vogalene

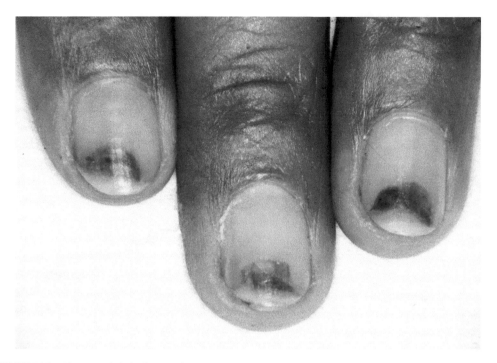

FIGURE 14.3   Photo-onycholysis due to a drug.

TABLE 14.3

Occupations Associated with Onycholysis

Barbers, beauticians	Laundry workers
Bartenders	Leather and pelt workers
Brewers	Manual laborers
Cigar makers	Milkers
Confectioners	Miners
Dish and bottle washers	Nut crackers
Domestic workers	Poultry pluckers
Farmers	Trauma
Gardeners	Typists
Housewives	Washerwomen

In fingernails, the most common causes come from trauma, cosmetic or occupational, and often onychotillomania (Figure 14.4). Maceration from prolonged immersion is often observed in women (Table 14.3).

Treatment

Successful therapy depends upon the elimination of exacerbating factors: above all maintaining fingernails at shorter lengths, using a hair blower once or twice a day, protecting the fingers with cotton-

TABLE 14.4

Onycholysis Due to Various Conditions

Infectious diseases	Dermatological conditions
Fungal disease	Alopecia areata
Dermatophytes	Congenital ectodermal defects
Non dermatophytes molds	Dermatitis
Yeast	Hyperhidrosis
Bacterial disease	Lichen planus
Corynebacterium	Lichen striatus
Leprosy	Onychotillomania
Proteus mirabilis	Pemphigus vegetans
Pseudomonas	Psoriasis
Syphilis	Subungual tumors
Viral disease	*Systemic conditions*
Herpes	Amyloidosis
Herpes zoster	Diabetes mellitus
Warts	Histiocytosis
Congenital and/or hereditary	Impaired circulation
Congenital toenail malalignment	Iron deficiency anemia
Hereditary Ectodermal dysplasias	Lung cancer
Epidermolysis bullosa	Lupus erythematosus
Onycholysis partialis (distal)	Mycosis fongoides
Pachyonychia congenita	Photoonycholysis
	Pellagra
	Porphyria
	Pregnancy
	Pseudo porphyria
	Raynaud's disease
	Scleroderma
	Shell nail syndrome
	Thyroid disease
	Yellow nail syndrome
Local causes	
New footwear, any trauma, orthopedic deformities (AGNUS)	

gloves beneath plastic or rubber-gloves. A more adapted treatment will be used according to the results demonstrated by culture on Sabouraud's media.

Treatment for onycholysis varies and depends on its cause. Eliminating and appropriately treating the predisposing cause of onycholysis is the best way. Treatment is unnecessary as photo-onycholysis disappears spontaneously. When the causes quoted in the tables are the culprits, prevention with dark nail varnish is recommended. Phototesting is negative.

Patients with onycholysis should be informed that cutting the nails as short as possible and avoiding trauma, contact with irritating or caustic products, and prolonged contact with water, is extremely important in dealing with their problem.

Patients should clip the affected portion of the nail and keep the nails short, and they should wear light cotton gloves under vinyl ones for any wet work.

Women patients can use colored nail varnish, first to cover the problem, and also to protect their nails from the possibility of photo-onycholysis, in case they use a medication which can cause such a condition. In the case of photo-onycholysis improvement of the nails is seen in 2–3 months and complete cure after almost 1 year.

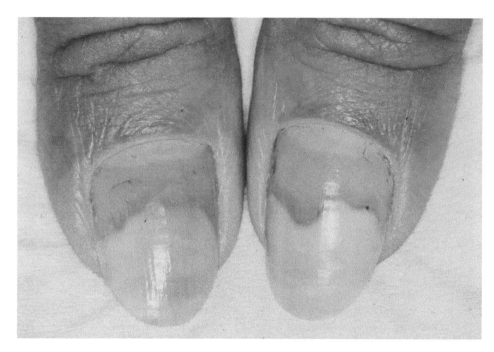

FIGURE 14.4   Mechanical onycholysis with advanced proximal margin.

Protection of the toe with a silicone cup is recommended.

Patients treated with docetaxel should wear frozen gloves (they contain glycerine which has thermal properties; it should be refrigerated for at least 3 hours, at 25°C–30°C). These should be used 15 minutes prior to the administration of the medication, during the infusion, and 15 minutes after the end of treatment.

Hard-palate mucosal graft has been used with success in long-standing idiopathic onycholysis. (Dominguez-Cherit and Daniel 2010).

BIBLIOGRAPHY

Baran R. (1986) Les onycholyses. *Ann Dermatol Venereol*; 113: 159–170.

Baran R., Mascaro J., Aguilera P. (2019) Photoonycholysis new findings. *JEADV*; 33: 56–62.

Daniel R., Tosti A., Iorizzo M, Piraccini B. M. (2017) The disappearing nail bed, a possible outcome of onycholysis. *Skin Appendage Disorders*; 3: 15–17.

Dominguez-Cherit J., Daniel R. C. (2010) Simple onycholysis an attempt at surgical intervention. *Dermatol Surg*; 36: 1791–1793.

Kechijian P. (1985) Onycholysis of the fingernail: Evaluation and management. *J Am Acad Dermatol*; 12: 552–560.

Zaias N., Escovar S. X., Zaias M. N. (2015) Finger and toenail onycholysis. *JEADV*; 20: 248–253.

15

Nail fragility and nail beautification

Robert Baran

Introduction

Nail beauty depends firstly upon nail health, but it is highly subjective, and evolving aspects of nail beauty are related to fashion.

The texture of the nail affects its appearance and function. Soft or brittle nails are obviously fragile. This results in unattractive longitudinal and horizontal splitting. Fragility is encouraged by wet work and excessive nail manicuring, especially the repeated application and removal of nail cosmetics. Critical to the esthetic appeal of the nail is its shape; most pleasing were the nails that conformed to the "magic ratio" in which the nail's length was approximately equal to its breadth, especially the thumb. The role of nail decoration and nail art in nail beauty is a subjective and evolving question of fashion, but for nails of equal length and corresponding contour, a painted nail is more attractive.

Besides its roles in cosmetic beauty, the nail also has a functional role. Both depend on three main factors: the shape of the nail, its decoration, and its texture.

A

BRITTLE NAIL OR NAIL FRAGILITY SYNDROME

Strength is the ability of the nail plate to withstand breakage

Stiffness/Rigidity/Hardness measures how easily the nail plate is scratched or indented.

Flexibility determines how much the plate will bend

Brittleness shows how likely the nail is to break

Toughness is a combination of strength and flexibility

Clinically, brittle nail syndrome encompasses six main types:

1. Onychorrhexis is made of shallow parallel furrows running in the superficial layer of the nail. It may result in an isolated split at the free edge, which sometimes extends proximally.

(a) 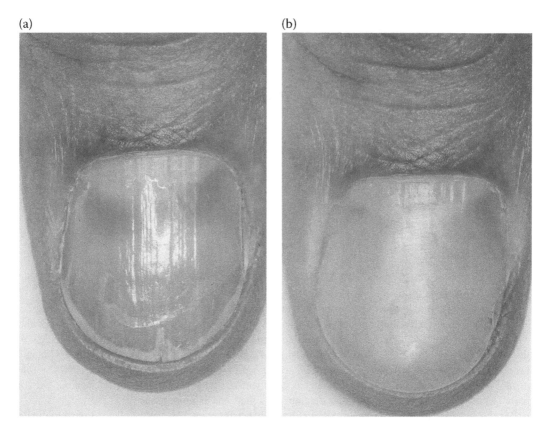 (b)

FIGURE 15.1   (a, b) Distal split of the nail.

2. A distal split Figure 15.1; a single longitudinal split involving the entire nail plate is sometimes observed (it may be produced by focal matrix Lichen planus).
3. Multiple, crenellated splitting.
4. Lamellar splitting of the free edge (Figure 15.2).
5. Transverse splitting and breaking of the lateral edge, usually close to the distal margin.

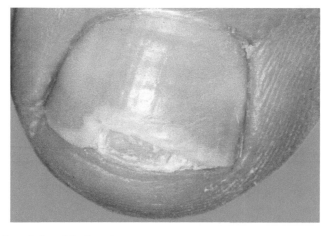

FIGURE 15.2   Lamellar splitting of the free edge.

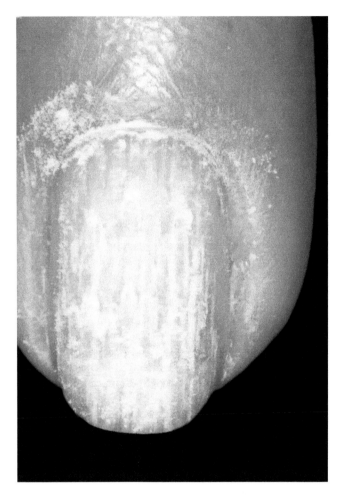

FIGURE 15.3 Nail keratin granulation partially abraded (pseudo leukonychia).

6. Friable nails were the changes are often confined to the surface of the nail plate. This often occurs in superficial onychomycosis or after application of nail polish causing "granulations" of the nail keratin which appear also spontaneously in psoriasis. They belong to the group of pseudo leukonychia (Figure 15.3).

According to causative factors we can distinguish two main forms of fragility: idiopathic and secondary to multiple causes.

- **Idiopathic nail fragility syndrome**
    Brittle nail syndrome is the most common cause. It is mainly observed in women, perhaps, because there is a decrease of cholesterol sulfate of the nail with age and probably the condition of their daily work at home.
- **Secondary nail fragility syndrome**
    Several inflammatory disorders are involved such as psoriasis, lichen planus, alopecia areata, Darier's disease, and eczema.
- **Infections**

Superficial white onychomycosis (but also distal type). Some diseases such as syphilis and pulmonary tuberculosis favor nail brittleness.

- **General conditions**

    Impairment of peripheral circulation secondary to arteriopathy, neurologic disorders, chronic anemia, aging, endocrine disorders (especially hypothyroidism), amyloidosis, chemotherapy, severe deficiency of vitamins trace elements, and amino acids from daily food intake.

- **Traumas**

    Most of them are occupational. In addition, onychotillomania and onychophagia play an important role.

    Finally, most of the techniques used to prepare "nail beauty" will contribute to weaken the nail.

Treatment of Brittle Nails

Most patients with brittle nails have an idiopathic nail fragility.

A combination with arginine silicate complex and magnesium biotinate was demonstrated to increase nail growth (Komorowsky et al. 2019*).

Iron supplementation (plus vitamin C) may be effective when ferritin levels are below 10 ng/ml (Iorizzo 2015).

As Zn deficiency is a cause of nail fragility prolonged treatment with zinc 20–30 mg/die seems to be effective (Di Baise and Parleton 2019).

A biomineral formulation containing amino-acids (L-cystine, L-arginine, glutamic acid), vitamins C, E, B6, B7) and mineral (zinc, iron, and copper) proved to be well tolerated and effective in improving fingernails in subjects with onychoschizia after 3 months of treatment (Sparavigna, Tenconi, and La Penna 2019)

Oral supplementation of bioactive collagen peptides was very effective: nail growth rate increased by 12% and the frequency of broken nails decreased by 42% (Hexel et al. 2017*).

Hydroxy propyl chitosan nail lacquer is useful to improve nail structure. (*Sparavigna et al. 2014*).

In recalcitrant nail fragility, nail wrapping limited to the distal portion of the nail may be useful (Baran and Andre 2005*).

Nail moisturizers are also useful in patients with brittle nails (Dahdah and Scher 2006*).

- Recognition of the causative agents and their elimination, whenever this is possible, is considered crucial for the management of onycholysis.
- Patients should keep their nails short, as long nail act as levers.
- They should also avoid contact with chemicals or physical agents that could harm them.
- Patients should wear cotton gloves under vinyl or nitrile one in any wet work.
- Do not use nails as tools or instruments.
- Spontaneous onycholysis, due to the sun does exist.

BIBLIOGRAPHY

Baran R., Andre J. (2005) Side effects of nail cosmetics. *J Cosmet Dermatol*; 4: 204–209.

Dahdah M. J., Scher R. K. (2006) Nail diseases related to nail cosmetics. *Dermatol Clin*; 24: 233–239.

Di Baise M., Parleton S. M. (2019) Hair, nails and skin: differentiating cutaneous manifestations of micronutrient deficiency. *Nutr Clin Pract*; 34: 490–503.

Hexel D., Zague V., Schunck M., Siega C., et al. (2017) Oral supplementation with specific bioactive collagen peptides improves nail growth and reduces symptoms of brittleness. *J Cosmet Dermatol*; 16: 5210–5216.

Iorizzo M. (2015) Tips to treat the five most common nail disorders: brittle nails, onycholysis, paronychia, psoriasis, onychomycosis. *Dermatol Clin*; 33: 175–178.

Komorowsky J., Perez Ojalvo S., Sylla S. et al. (2019) The effect of combination of an Arginine Silicate Complex and Magnesium Biotinate on hair and nail growth in rats (PO6-026-19). *Curr Dev Nutr*; 3 (Suppl 1): nzz031.P06-026-19.

Sparavigna A., Caserini M., Tenconi B., et al. (2014) Effects of a novel nail lacquer based on hydroxypropyl Chitosan (HPCH) in subjects with finger nail onychoschizia). *J Dermatol Clin Res*; 2: 1013–1018.

Sparavigna A., Tenconi B., La Penna L. (2019) Efficacy and tolerability of a biomineral formulation for treatment of onychoschizia: randomized trial. *Clin Cosmet Investing Dermtol*; 13: 355–362.

B

PREVENTATIVE MEASURES IN CASE OF NAIL FRAGILITY

- Keep nails short.
- Limit contact with water.
- Detergents are forbidden.
- Use cotton gloves under plastic or nitrile gloves.
- After any soaking apply topical moisturizers.
- Avoid manicuring with sharp tools.
- Leave cuticles uncut.
- Artificial nails should be avoided.

Formaldehyde Nail Hardeners

Reactions to nail hardeners are well recognized. They are usually attributed to their formaldehyde content.

However, the INCI dictionary no longer requires manufacturers to call formalin by the incorrect name formaldehyde. Formaldehyde is an anhydrous gas that upon mixing with water reacts to form a methylene glycol and residual traces of formaldehyde in equilibrium.

Most products never exceed 1.5% methylene glycol since at higher concentrations. Both the nail plate and the surrounding tissue can quickly show signs of adverse changes. At these concentrations, used products contain less than 12 ppm (0.0012%) free formaldehyde. Companies selling these products generally disregard requirements for skin shields, so accidental skin exposure can occur. Using a concentration of less than 0.2% methylene glycol seems to have little or to no positive benefits on the surface hardness of the nail plate.

The nail changes previously reported are onycholysis, nail discoloration, subungual hemorrhages, subungual hyperkeratosis, and dryness of the skin. Discontinuation of the nail Hardener resulted in complete resolution of the nail dystrophy. Another abnormality painful thickening of the hyponychium (pterygium inversum unguis) may follow the inappropriate use of nail "fortifier" with formaldehyde.

The distal part of the nail bed remains adherent to the ventral surface of the nail plate. The distal groove is then obliterated. The pain associated with this disorder is probably due to traction on the nail neurovascular network underlying the hyponychium.

Though positive patch tests to formaldehyde have been elicited in some patients, other workers have suggested that it is an irritant rather than an allergic contact reaction.

As a rule, use of formaldehyde is no longer allowed on the market.

FURTHER READING

Fisher A., Baran R. (1992) Occupational nail disorders with a reference to Koebner phenomenon. *Am J Contact Dermatitis*; 3: 16–23.

Schoon D., Baran R. (2017) Cosmetics for Abnormal and Pathological Nails. In *Textbook of Cosmetic Dermatology*. 5th ed. CRC Press.

C

GEL NAIL POLISH

Gel polish, also known as ultra violet curable nail lacquer, has gained popularity for its cosmetic enhancement, long-lasting duration, resistance to chipping, denting, scratching, and its easy application.

Gel polish contains a base of 75%–95% urethane (meth) acrylate oligomers and cross-linking monomers 1%–4% polymerization photoinitiators and 0.75%–1.25% catalysts such as dimethyl tolylamine.

Unfortunately, "Gel polish has been documented to cause pincer nail deformities, yellowish chromonychia, nail thinning paronychia, pseudoleukonychia, onychoschizia, lamellar splitting, allergic contact dermatitis and psoriasiform nail changes" (Cervantes et al. 2018).

In addition, pterygium inversum unguis may appear characterized by the abnormal adherence of the hyponychium to the ventral surface of the nail plate, an area unsightly and painful (Cervantes et al. 2018).

BIBLIOGRAPHY

Cervantes J., Sanchez M., Eber A. E. et al. (2018) Pterygium inversum unguis secondary to gel polish. *JEADV*; 32: 160–163.

D

Gel nail polish and loss of all fingernails

Each coat nails were subjected to UV light for 30 sec. One week after, the nails started to peel off, and this was associated with pain, and they shed off completely.

Two weeks later: the nails started to regrow and the time of presentation physical exam showed re-growth proximal part of the nail plate and brown hyperpigmentation of the distal nail bed (Alwash and Gupta 2018).

BIBLIOGRAPHY

Alwash N., Gupta P. (2018) A case of complete loss of fingernails following application of gel nail polish. *Br J Dermatol*; 179 (suppl 1): 96.

E

Acrylic nail (porcelain nail) paresthesia

Pain and persistent paresthesia have been reported in a dental nurse, but permanent paresthesia may occur without an allergic reaction. Paronychial inflammation may be quite severe: dentist's occupational allergic paronychia associated with fingertip dermatitis can be caused by acrylics. In some cases, sensitization may produce significant economic and mental stress in affected patients. Interestingly, no difference in the occurrence of skin problems was observed between individuals using gloves and individuals who did not use gloves while handling acrylates. Nail discoloration may occur and the nail bed itself usually becomes dry and thickened. Onycholysis of the natural nail occurs with thinning and splitting. This disfiguration of the nail plate can last for many months. Loss of fingernails due to persisting allergic contact dermatitis in an artificial gel nail designer is rarely reported.

BIBLIOGRAPHY

Baran R., Schibli H. (1990) Permanent paresthesia to sculptured nails: a distressing problem. *Dermatol. Clin.*; 8: 139–141.
Kanerva L., Mikola H., Enricks-Eckerman M. L., et al. (1998) Fingertip paresthesia and occupational allergic contact dermatitis caused by acrylics in a dental nurse. *Contact Dermatitis*; 38: 114–116.

F

Powder gel nail (dipped nails, dipping powders)

The **powder gel nail enhancement system** has fewer allergic reactions than the older acrylics (due to monomers) and the gel shellac systems that use UV or LED light to polymerize the product.

The gel powder systems (sometimes called dip powder gels) begin with cyanoacrylate basecoat, followed immediately by acrylate powder dusted or dipped onto the wet base. An aqueous catalyst is brushed on top to harden the powder. The powder is identical to the old acrylic nail polymer powder but safer because the allergenic monomer is not used. In fact, all nail enhancement systems damage the nail plate. Application of all artificial nail systems begins with buffing or filing, the surface of the nail plate. This damaging procedure is performed every 3 weeks when the new product is reapplied. Not surprisingly, the free edge of the nail plate becomes very thin and brittle after 4–6 months of this activity. Allergic reactions are less problematic with the powder systems but when it happens, cyanoacrylate in the base coat is always the culprit *(Rich P., Personal communication).*

G

PREFORMED ARTIFICIAL NAILS

Plastic press-on nails are preformed and glued to the nail with cyanoacrylate preparation. They are packaged in several shapes and sizes to conform to normal nail plate configurations. They are used as full nails or nail tips, fixed with a special adhesive, supplied with the kit. Preformed nails in gold plate may be used in the same way as plastic nails. The application of preformed prosthetic nails is limited by the need for some normal nail to be present for attachment. Some manufacturers recommend that they should not remain on for more than one or two days at a time.

Artificial tips are the primary application of prosthetic nails. Most nail technicians feel it is too time-consuming to sculpt nails. Therefore, they use acrylic tips and overlays.

Preformed nails remaining in place for more than three or four days can cause onycholysis and nail surface damage.

Allergic onychia and paronychia due to cyanoacrylate nail preparations may be observed. After about three months, painful paronychia, onychia, dystrophy, and discoloration of the nails may become apparent and last for several months. Eyelid dermatitis disappears with removal of the allergen.

H

NAIL MENDING AND WRAPPING

The purpose of nail mending is to create a splint for a partially fractured nail plate or one split extending the full length of the nail. The split is first bonded with cyanoacrylate monomer. Then a piece of wrap fabric is cut and shaped to fit over the nail surface. This is then embedded within the cyanoacrylate monomer and several coats are applied; or the fabric is applied directly over the crack and subsequently sealed to nail with cyanoacrylate monomer, or no-light gel. In nail wrapping or "wraps", the free edge of the nail should be long enough to be splinted with paper, silk, linen, or fiberglass and fixed to the plate with cyanoacrylate monomer. The activator for cyanoacrylate wraps is a catalyst and contains N,N-dimethyl-toluidine in a solvent carrier. Methemoglobinemia with resultant cyanosis may follow its ingestion. DMPT is typically 0.5% of the formulation and HQ up to 1000 ppm. The ethyl acetate and trichloroethane in these products do not promote curing, but are instead solvents.

Paper is not very effective, but silk wraps are sheer, very thin, and work quite well. Linen is thicker and offers increased strength but inhibits cyanoacrylate penetration to the nail, thus, lowering adhesion and does not have as natural an appearance as other materials. Fiberglass combines many benefits of both silk and linen and is the most universally used.

Most wrap systems consist of a few basic elements.

Monomeric cyanoacrylate, polymerizing from moisture in the air or in the natural nail's surface, to form the hard nail coating that is both the base and top coats of the nail wrap.

A mesh material, for example, fiberglass or silk, is preferred.

An activator or catalyst cuts the hardening time to seconds.

16

Nail prostheses

Annie Pillet
Robert Baran

In a wide variety of distal phalanx cases, ranging from a nail deformation, loss of tissue, to a complete loss of the distal phalanx, a short silicone prosthesis, known as a "thimble" prosthesis (Pillet and Didierjean-Pillet 2001) makes it possible to leave the **D**istal **I**nter-**P**halangeal area free (Figures 16.1, 16.2, 16.3, 16.4) Even ectrodactyly can benefit from the prothesis technique (Figures 16.5, 16.6).

This digital prosthesis is made of silicone and fits the stump perfectly.

The prosthesis should restore the volume and shape of the finger, from an esthetic point of view, as well as the texture of the skin and the striates. The color should be indistinguishable from the supporting finger.

It must be flexible and thin enough in order to allow mobility of the articulations and ensure that the limit between prosthesis and the supporting finger is as inconspicuous as possible.

The "thimble" prosthesis permits modification of the consistency of the pulp, along with being relatively flexible in order to increase surface contact.

The prosthetic nail is cosmetic. It supports the use and removal of nail polish.

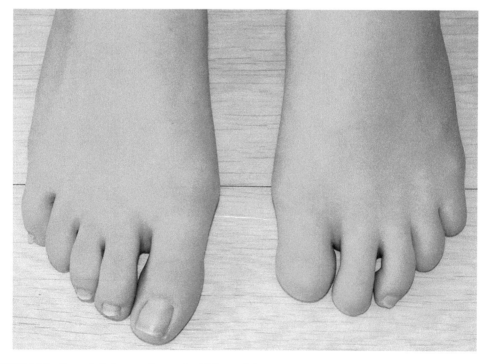

FIGURE 16.1   Congenital absence of some distal left toe phalanges.

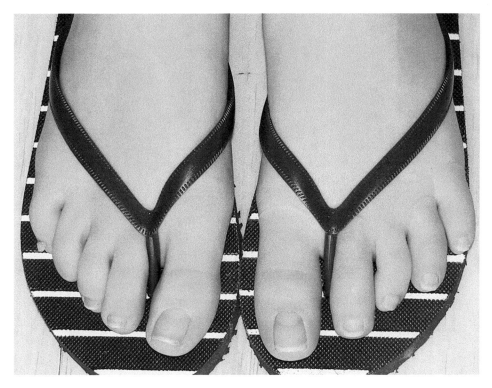

FIGURE 16.2   Same patient with prosthetic substitution.

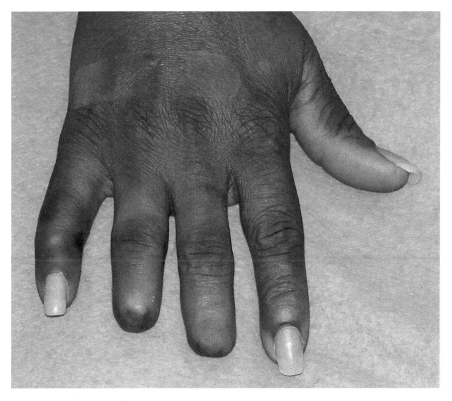

FIGURE 16.3   Traumatic partial amputation of two distal phalanges.

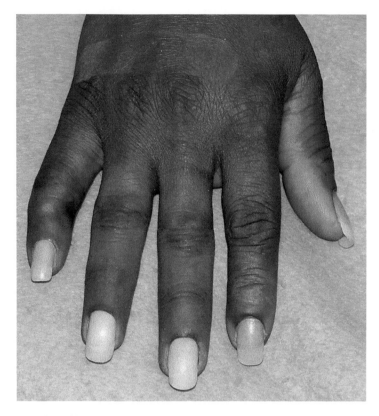

FIGURE 16.4   Same patient with prosthetic substitution.

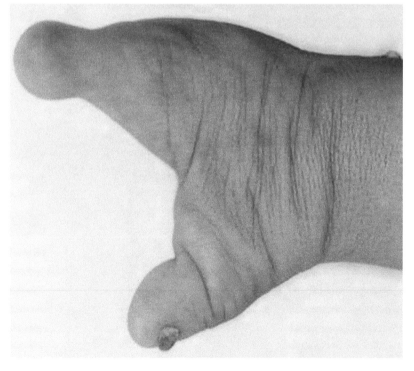

FIGURE 16.5   Ectrodactyly.

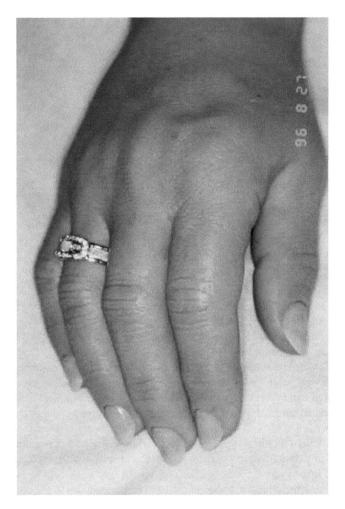

FIGURE 16.6 Same patient with prosthetic substitution.

Two types of prosthesis exist:

* A rigid fingernail which is the most frequently used, or
* A flexible fingernail, the technique of which is at present very advanced. Today, this technique finds its only application in certain very specific long stump cases.

BIBLIOGRAPHY

Beasley R. W., de Bez G. (1990) Prosthetic substitution for fingernail. *Hand Clinic*; 6: 105–112.
Pillet J., Didierjean-Pillet A. (2001) Ungual prosthesis. *J. Dermatol Treatment*; 12: 41–46.

17

Nail pigmentation

Robert Baran
Dimitris Rigopoulos

Drugs

Periungual hyperpigmentation in newborns is a physiological melanic pigmentation observed during the early months of life. In addition, several types of acro pigmentation have been described in pediatric nail disorders (Baran, Hadj-Rabia, and Silverman 2017). In adults one has to rule out Hutchinson's sign (Figure 17.1) from nonmelanoma Hutchinson's sign.

Pigmentation of the nails caused by medications can be of melanocytic or nonmelanocytic origin. When a drug activates the melanocytes of the nail matrix, the melanocytes may only be partially activated, and as such only a group of matrix melanocytes are activated to produce pigment, and a longitudinal pigmented band known as melanonychia results. Less commonly, this drug-induced melanocyte activation results in the appearance of pigmented transverse bands, alternating with bands of normal color.

Nail pigmentation caused by melanocyte activation leading to melanin deposition in the nail plate is a frequent side effect of chemotherapeutic agents doxorubicin, bleomycin, cyclophosphamide, daunorubicin, dacarbazine, hydroxyurea, methotrexate, and vincristine. Polydactylic melanonychia was induced by the topical applications of 5-fluorouracil on periungual warts affecting only two fingers.

TABLE 17.1

Adverse Drug Reactions in Nails

Affected area	Symptoms
Matrix	Nail fragility
	Beau's lines/ onychomadesis
	True leukonychia
	Melanonychia
Nail bed	Onycholysis
	Photo-onycholysis
	Apparent leukonychia
	Dermal pigmentation
	Hemorrhagic onycholysis
Nail folds	Paronychia
	Pyogenic granuloma
	Newborn's periungual hyperpigmentation
	Hutchinson's sign
	Nonmelanoma Hutchinson's sign

Source: From Adigun 2016. With permission.

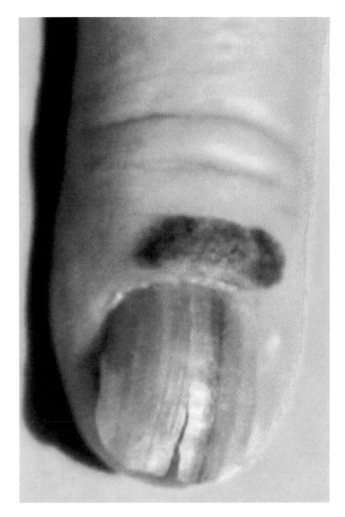

FIGURE 17.1   Hutchinson's sign.

This pigmentation involving the lunula of the nails of all fingers was identical to that induced by systemically administered cytotoxic drugs, recalling the nail pigmentation following eye drops such as timolol maleate, a betablocker responsible for nail pigmentation (Baran and Laugier 1985).

Another unexpected side effect of topical 5FU appeared in a 68-year-old man treating an actinic keratosis on his right temple nightly for 1 month. He was seen 2 weeks after he had ceased treatment and showed brown discoloration of his left-hand fingernails. It turned out that he usually slept on his right side with his left hand tucked under his face (Callander and Jong 2015). Nail plate – nail bed separation has been reported in systemic 5FU administration (Katz and Hansen 1979) and yellow nails in the topical treatment of nail psoriasis (Fiallo 2012).

Transverse pigmented bands caused by intermittent melanin production can be seen with psoralen with ultraviolet A, infliximab, and zidovudine, as well as the synthetic Melanotan injections.

Non melanocytic pigmentation caused by medications has a different pathogenesis, deposition of pigments in the dermis of the periungual region. Minocycline has been reported to cause nails to appear a blue-gray color, but typically spares the lunula (Geria et al. 2009). A blue, brown, or grey pigmentation that does not move distally with growth can be seen in patients treated with long-term antimalarial therapy (Kalabalikis et al. 2010). Zidovudine causes a characteristic blue or brown hyperpigmentation of the nails, with blue lunulae and/or dark brown nail plates (Piraccini and Tosti 1999). Azure nails are classically described in silver toxicity.

(a)   (b)

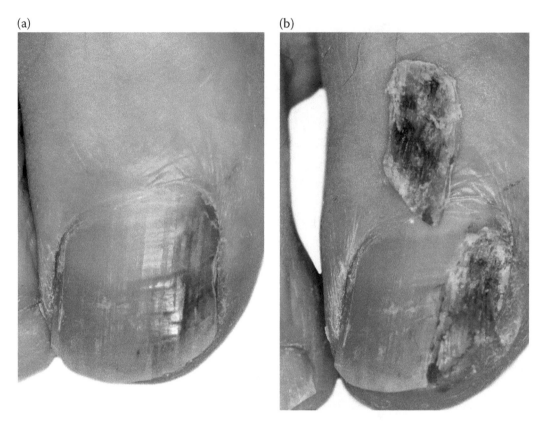

FIGURE 17.2   (a, b) *Trichophyton rubrum nigricans.*

Fungal Infections

Fungal infections may cause nail plate pigmentation either by melanocytic activation or by melanin pigmentation produced by the fungus itself.

*Some strains of **dermatophytes*** may produce a soluble, non-granular melanin that stains the nail plate brown to black (Figure 17.2a-b). Histopathology shows a diffuse yellowish-brown pigmentation of the nail substance and also fungal hyphae in the subungual keratotic debris. This melanin may be either Fontana-Masson argentaffin positive or negative.

Black molds such as *Neoscytalidium dimidiatum, Aspergillus niger, Exophiala, Wangiella* spp., and *Alternaria alternata* usually cause a more diffuse brown nail pigmentation. Their cell walls contain melanin, and this can be confirmed in a Fontana-Masson stain.

A distolateral onychomycosis due to *Phialophora* spp. was reported in a 77-year-old male presenting with a blackish-brown longitudinal pigmentation of the nail plate of the right index spreading onto the proximal nail fold.

Candida Infection

One diabetic patient developed hyperpigmentation of the nail unit including nail plate and periungual tissues in conjunction with a culture-proven *Candida albicans* (Figure 17.3a,b) and *C. parapsilosis* (Figure 17.4a,b) infection. Hyperpigmentation cleared following avulsion and topical antifungal therapy.

(a) (b)

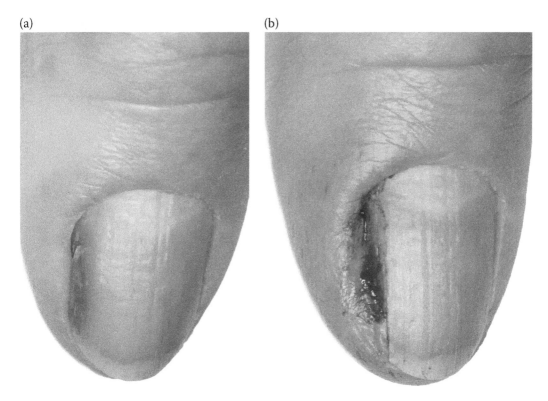

FIGURE 17.3 (a, b) *Candida albicans.*

(a) (b)

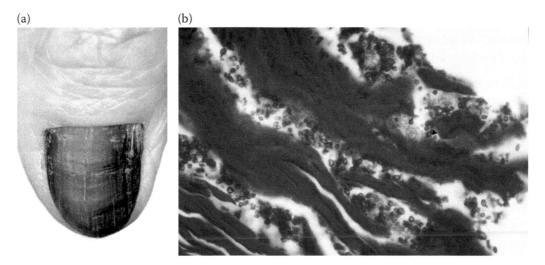

FIGURE 17.4 (a, b) *Candida parapsilosis.*

Bacterial Pigmentation

Most bacteria producing a gray to black pigment belong to the group of Gram-negative pathogens, most commonly *Klebsiella* and *Proteus mirabilis*. The latter causes a dark green pigmentation that usually originates under the junction of the lateral and proximal nail folds or in the lateral nail groove and may

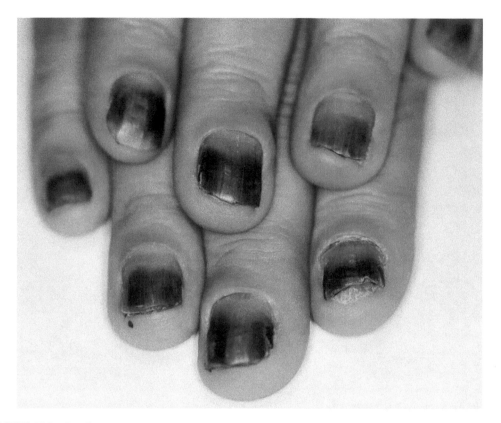

FIGURE 17.5   *Pseudomonas aeruginosa.*

eventually spread over most of the nail plate. Green nails are exceptionally found in isolation. They may be associated with nail plate–nail bed separation (Bauer and Cohen 1957; Chernosky and Dukes 1963).

The nails may be a part of the triad characterizing the "green nail" syndrome: (1) a greenish discoloration of the nail plate (Figure 17.5); (2) paronychia; and (3) *Pseudomonas* infection with onycholysis and fruity odor frequently observed.

Pseudomonas may be isolated in culture, but it often happens that the culture does not yield any bacteria. The colors vary from a light green to dark green/black. *Pseudomonas* species produce a number of different diffusible pigments, such as pyocyanin (dark green) and fluorescein (yellow-green). Both are soluble in water and the former is also soluble in chloroform. Green transverse striped nails may result from repeated episodes of bacterial infection of the proximal nail fold, with deposition of organisms and pigment during each episode. The differential diagnosis of green nail syndrome includes:

- Dark green pigmentation with *Proteus mirabilis* (Quadripur, Schauder, and Schwartz 2001). This Gram-negative bacillus generates hydrogen sulfide. This compound reacts with traces of metals in the nail plate, such as zinc, nickel, cobalt, iron, manganese, tin, copper, and lead metal sulfides, to blacken the nail plate. The disappearance of the blackening is observed after topical treatment with chinosol, iodine, and chloramphenicol solution.

- Light greenish discoloration sometimes observed in psoriasis is due to serum glycoproteins but associated *Pseudomonas* infection can also be diagnosed using Wood's lamp that produces fluorescence.

- Green nail discoloration also may be secondary to use of the antiseptic "brilliant green," a bactericidal (triphenylmethane dye) and may cause blindness with eye contact (Chelidze 2020).

- At present, it is not believed with certitude that either *Candida* spp. or *Aspergillus* is responsible for the green hue.
- While others advocate the use of oral antibiotics, such as ciprofloxacin, we consider crucial keeping the nails dry and correcting any environmental factors, such as excessive wet work or manicuring. A drop of sodium hypochlorite solution (Milton™) applied twice a day has a beneficial effect on the discoloration. Onycholytic portion of the nail can be removed and nail bed treated with antiseptics such as 2% acetic acid.

Black nail may be seen through the plate by transparency in a rare syndrome, *Purpura fulminans*, a serious complication of varicella infection.

BIBLIOGRAPHY

Adigun C. G. (2016) Adverse drugs reactions of the lower extremities. *Clin Podiatr Med Surg*; 33: 397–408.

Baran R., Laugier P. (1985) Melanonychia induced by topical 5-fluouracil. *Br J Dermatol*; 112: 621–625.

Baran R., Hadj-Rabia S., Silverman R (2017) *Pediatric Nail Disorders*, Chapter 5. CRC Press.

Bauer M. F., Cohen B. A. (1957) The role of Pseudomonas in infection about the nails. *Arch Dermatol*; 75: 394–396.

Callander J., Jong C (2015) An unexpected side-effect of topical 5FU. *Br J Dermatol*; 173 (suppl S1): 88.

Chelidze K, Lipner S (2020) Brilliant green staining of the fingernails. *Cutis*; 105: 317–318.

Chernosky M, Dukes D (1963) Green nails. *Arch Dermatol*; 88: 548–553.

Fiallo P (2012) Yellow nails as an adverse reaction to the topical use of 5-FU for the treatment of nail psoriasis. *J Dermatol Treat*; 23: 82–89.

Geizals S, Lipner SR (2020) Retrospective case series on risk factors, diagnosis and treatment of pseudomonas aeruginosa nail infections. *Am J Clin Dermatol*; 21: 297–302.

Geria AN, Tajirian AL, Kihiczak G et al. (2009) Minocycline-induced skin pigmentation: an update. *Acta Dermatovenereol Croat*; 17 (2): 123–126.

Kalabalikis D, Patsatsi A, Trakatelli MG et al. (2010) Hyperpigmented forearms and nail: a quiz. *Acta Derm Venereol*; 90(6): 657–659.

Katz ME, Hansen TW (1979) Nail plate-nail bed separation. An unusual side-effect of systemic fluorouracil administration. *Arch Dermatol*; 115: 860–861.

Piraccini BM, Tosti A (1999) Drug-induced nail disorders: incidence management and prognosis. *Drug Saf*; 21(3): 187–201.

Quadripur SA, Schauder S, Schwartz P (2001) Black nails from *Proteus mirabilis* colonisation. *Hautarzt*; 52: 658–661.

Romaszkiewicz A, Stawinska M, Sojanek M, Nowichi RJ (2018) Nail dermoscopy (onychoscopy) is useful in diagnosis and treatment follow-up of the nail mixed infection caused by *Pseudomonas aeruginosa* and *Candida albicans*. *Postepy Dermatol Alergol*; 35: 327–329.

18

How to prevent and treat chemotherapy-induced nail abnormalities

Richard Encaoua

Cytotoxic chemotherapies, targeted therapies, and immunotherapies can induce nail changes.

These nail toxicities are common for patients during the course of cancer treatment (Robert et al. 2015; Sibaud et al. 2016). A study carried out in a French cancer center revealed that among the patients who received these anticancer agents and had dermatological adverse events, 39% had nail changes (Robert et al., 2015).

More specifically, cytotoxic chemotherapy more frequently produces toxic effects on the nail. A prospective Indian study found nail changes in 71.3% of patients on chemotherapy. The most represented cancer was breast cancer (39.5%) and taxanes the molecule most often responsible (Zawar et al. 2019).

Most frequently changes in **chemotherapy** affect the nail plate and the nail bed:

- Changes in pigmentation like melanonychia with cyclophosphamide, doxorubicin and hydroxyurea, true leukonychia with cyclophosphamide, doxorubicin, and vincristine, and also apparent leukonychia.
- But changes can also affect transitory decrease of matrix activity leading to Beau's lines (Figure 18.1) or onychomadesis and reducing the nail growth and thickness.
- Other modifications occurred like onycholysis and hematomas principally, with taxanes and could sometimes complicated with secondary infection, most of the time with *Pseudomonas aeruginosa*, causing green or yellow coloration and suppuration.

On the other hand, toxic effects to the periungual tissue, paronychia and pyogenic granuloma lesions, are more frequent with targeted treatments like **EGFR inhibitors (EGFRIs)** and less frequently with **mTOR** and **MEK inhibitors**. Among EGFRIs, cetuximab is the most commonly reported cause (Figure 18.2) but new selective tyrosine kinase inhibitors are recently described (Garden et al., 2012; Lacouture 2019).

Immunotherapies are becoming more prevalent in clinical use in patients with cancers.

Autoimmune skin, hair, and mucosal disorders are frequently described in patients treated with these drugs like **checkpoint inhibitors** (monoclonal antibodies targeting cytotoxic T lymphocyte-associated antigen-4 (CTLA-4) or programmed cell death protein 1 (PD-1) (5).

Patients presenting with alopecia areata with nail changes were reported with monotherapy with checkpoint inhibitor (Figures 18.3, 18.4). Trachyonychia, onychoschizia, and distal onycholysis were the clinical forms most often described (Zarbo et al. 2017).

If nail unit toxicities induced by systemic drugs have been extensively reported, there are some papers recording unilateral nail unit changes related with anticancer therapies. This phenomenon has an explanation: the acral drug-induced toxicities require the integrity of the central and peripheral nervous system. This asymmetric acral phenomenon has been observed with taxanes, sorafenib, and adriamycin (Baran et al. 2018).

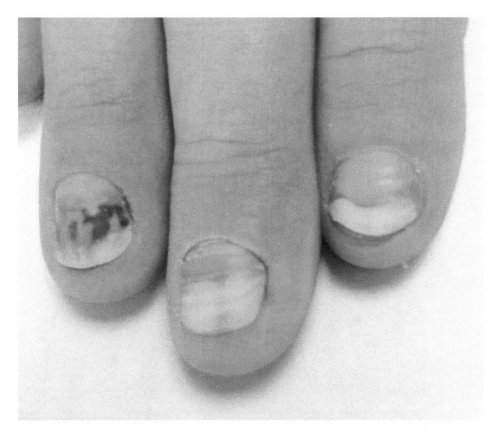

FIGURE 18.1 Onycholysis and Beau's lines with chemotherapy (taxanes).

All of the changes of the nail unit can be associated with pain and functional impairment which affect patient's quality of life.

Most anticancer drug-induced nail lesions do not require treatment as they are asymptomatic. Moreover, at the time of diagnosis they reflect the past effects of anticancer drugs on the matrix. Thus, changes like Beau's lines, onycholysis and pigmentation will disappear with nail growth and discontinuation of treatment. The nail will return to a normal appearance after its complete growth in 4 to 6 months for hands and 12 to 18 months for toes.

Furthermore, the patients can be advised about preventative measures to limit nail toxicities (nail plate changes, onycholysis and periungual lesions) (Robert et al. 2015; Lacouture 2015):

- Keep fingernails as dry as possible.
- Always use a double pair of gloves (first in cotton and second in vinyl, nitrile, or latex).
- Avoid repeated trauma or friction from manicuring and restrict frequent use of nail polish and nail polish removers.
- Use wide and comfortable shoes.
- Apply topical emollients to cuticles and periungual tissues frequently.
- Some nail lacquers such as hydroxypropyl chitosan or polyurethane 16% seem to be useful to reduce water evaporation from the nail plate and have a barrier effect
- Collaboration with a podiatrist can be useful.

A non-controlled study suggests the use of oral biotin or vitamin E.

A colored varnish may be recommended to mask abnormal nail coloration.

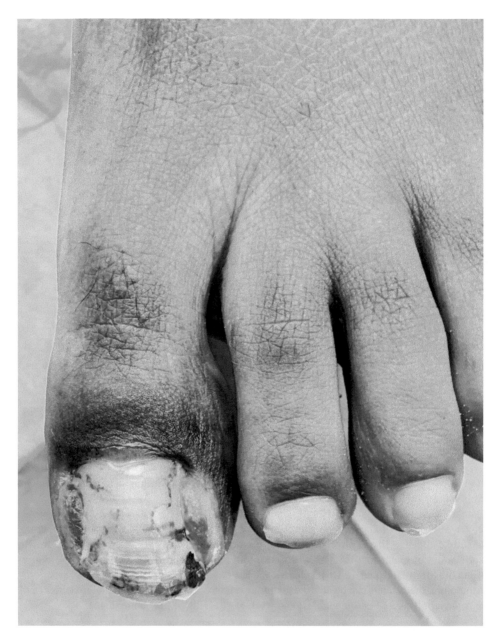

FIGURE 18.2   Bilateral pyogenic granuloma on toe with EGFR inhibitors (cetuximab).

The simple gesture of debridement of onycholysis allows immediate control of the pain in cases with or without underlying abscess or hematomas. Thereafter, the use of antiseptic solution to clean nail bed or a local antibiotic like mupirocin or fusidic acid helps to treat a possible infection.

For paronychia lesions and to prevent secondary infection, antiseptic solutions are used daily. Podiatrists can correct nail curvature if needed. To reduce the inflammation responsible for the pain, high-class of topical steroids alone or in combination with topical antibiotics (fucidic acid or mupirocin) are prescribed. Other suggested modalities include intralesional injection of triamcinolone acetonide, followed by antiseptic lotion twice daily. Some positive response has been reported with the application of topical calcineurin inhibitors but also with the use of oral tetracyclines. Finally, in cases with clinical signs of infection, microbiological samples will will help advise appropriate oral antibiotic treatment.

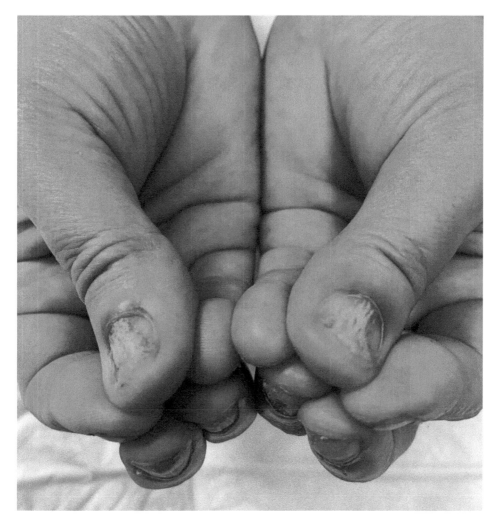

FIGURE 18.3   Nail changes with immunotherapy (checkpoint inhibitors); alopecia areata was also observed.

Pyogenic granuloma lesions are more difficult to manage. In case of severe pain, several affected digits and if the patient's quality of life is affected, a reduction in the dose, a temporary interruption or the discontinuation of treatment may be offered. Indeed, these lesions often depend on the dose and regress in the event of modification.

Before these adjustments of anticancer treatment, topical application of liquid nitrogen, topical steroids or weekly 10% aqueous silver nitrate, 35% trichloroacetic acid or phenol 88% applications as well as topical beta-blockers (timolol and propranolol) can be used to reduce granulation tissue.

Nevertheless, the standard of care for pyogenic granuloma is surgery when necessary. Under local digital block anesthesia, a curettage of granulation tissue and partial removal of the nail plate were completed with partial matricectomy confined to the lateral horns, achieved with chemical cauterization with 88% phenol (phenolization).

Conclusion

Nail toxicities are very frequent and varied in patients treated with chemotherapies, targeted therapies and immunotherapies. Easy preventive measures and guidelines should be prescribed because these

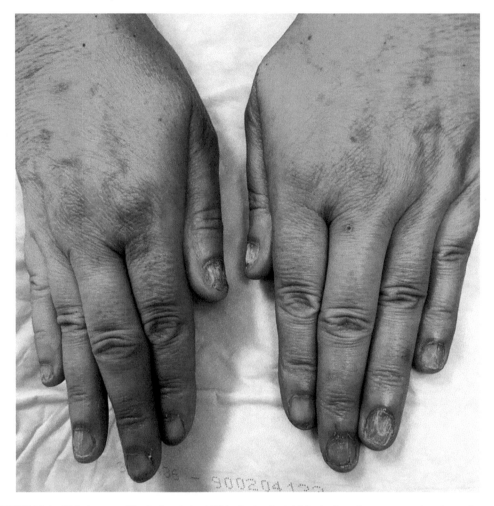

FIGURE 18.4   Nail changes with nivolumab (anti-PD1, checkpoint inhibitor); alopecia areata was also observed.

changes can affect patient's quality of life. Dermatologists must be trained in the medical and surgical management of these different anomalies in order to be able to respond with appropriate care to the different requests concerning these patients.

BIBLIOGRAPHY

Baran R, Robert C, Sibaud V (2018) Asymmetric Acral spared phenomenon related to systemic anticancer therapies. *Skin Appendage Disorders*; 4: 315–319.

Garden BC, Wu S, Lacouture ME (2012) The risk of nail changes with epidermal growth factor receptor inhibitors: a systemic review of the literature and meta-analysis. *J Am Acad Dermatol*; 67(3): 400–408.

Lacouture ME (2015) Management of dermatologic toxicities. *J Natl Compr Canc Netw*; 13 (suppl 5): 680–689.

Lacouture ME, Sibaud V (2018) Toxic side effects of targeted therapies and immunotherapies affecting the skin, oral mucosa, and nails. *American Journal of Clinical Dermatology*; 19(suppl 1): 31–39.

Robert C, Sibaud V, Mateus C et al. (2015) Nails toxicities induced by systemic anticancer treatments. *Lancet Oncol*; 16(4): e181–e189.

Sibaud V, Lebœuf NR, Roche H et al. (2016) Dermatological adverse events with taxane chemotherapy. *Eur J Dermatol*; 26(5): 427–443.

Zarbo A, Belum VR, Sibaud V et al. (2017) Immune-related alopecia (areata and universalis) in cancer patients receiving immune chekpoint inhibitors. *Br. J Dermatol*; 176(6): 1649–1652.

Zawar V, Bondarde S, Pawar M et al. (2019) Nails changes due to chemotherapy: a prospective observational study of 129 patients. *J Eur Acad Dermatol Venereol*; 33: 1398–1404.

19

Intralesional nail therapies

Chander Grover
Geetali Kharghoria

Introduction

The complex anatomy of the nail unit makes it a unique appendage. The germinative matrix is the core of the nail plate formation. It is guarded above by the impervious nail plate and the proximal nail fold, which is itself a fold of skin, thus forming a double epithelial barrier. The nail bed, also known as the sterile matrix, also contributes to some extent to nail plate formation and to its appearance. This too is protected by a thicker, more impervious nail plate (Figure 19.1). Both the nail matrix and nail bed are affected by various dermatoses like psoriasis, lichen planus and, in addition, disorders specific to nail epithelia including onychomycosis, subungual warts, trachyonychia, and nail unit tumors.

Topical drugs, which are useful in treatment of cutaneous or nail fold disease, are rendered ineffective in nail manifestations due to barriers in drug penetration. Similar constraints are encountered by systemic drugs like orally administered antifungals. Even if the systemically systemically adminstered antimicrobial drug is able to achieve minimal inhibitory concentrations in blood, the same may not hold true for the nail epithelia or the nail plate where the distorted architecture prevents effective drug diffusion from the nail bed. This leads to a failure to eradicate fungal colonization from the less vascular nail plate, which also acquires air spaces due to onychomycosis.

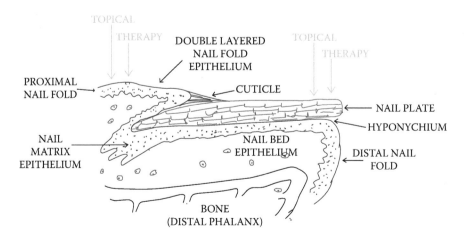

FIGURE 19.1 Sagittal anatomy of the nail unit showing barriers to penetration of topical therapy into the nail matrix epithelium or nail bed epithelium.

TABLE 19.1

Summary of Indications Where Injectable Therapy Has Been Used in Nails

Disease	Site/Type of injection	Drugs used	Dose	Interval
Nail psoriasis/ Acrodermatitis continua of Hallopeau	Nail matrix / Nail bed or hyponychium	Triamcinolone acetonide (TA) (2.5–10 mg/mL), can be diluted with 1% lidocaine without epinephrine or normal saline)	0.1 (depending on the size of the nail); Usually started with 5 mg/mL; May be reduced to 2.5 mg/mL over time	• Optimum 4-weekly for a minimum of 4–6 months (methotrexate injections have been administered more frequently)
		Methotrexate (25 mg/mL)	0.1 mL	
		Cyclosporine (50 mg/mL)	0.1 mL	• Followed by once every 6–8 weeks
Nail lichen planus	Nail matrix/ Nail bed (less commonly used)	TA (2.5–10 mg/mL)	0.1 mL	• Every 2 months for the final 6- to 12-month period
Trachyonychia	Nail matrix	TA (2.5–10 mg/mL)	0.1 mL	• Interval can be reduced in case of flare
Periungual/ subungual wart	Translesional/ Intralesional	Bleomycin (1–3 U/mL) [1U=1mg]. Like TA, this too can be diluted with local anesthetic to decrease the pain during injection	Injection into each and every wart (Maximum dose: 2 mg/session)	Fortnightly, till the lesion completely regresses
	Intralesional into larger warts (maximum of two warts per session)	Vitamin D3 (15 mg/mL)	0.1–0.2 mL(Max. 0.4 mL/session)	Fortnightly × 4 sessions or complete resolution (whichever is earlier)
	Intralesional into the single largest wart	MMR vaccine	0.1–0.5 mL	2–4 weekly × 3–5 sessions or complete resolution (whichever is earlier)
	Intralesional in a single wart	Mw (MIP) vaccine	0.1 mL	2–4 weekly × 10 sessions or complete resolution (whichever is earlier)
	Intralesional injection into the largest wart	Tuberculin purified protein derivative (PPD)	0.1 mL (10 IU)	Fortnightly × 6 sessions or complete resolution (whichever is earlier)
Myxoid pseudocyst	Translesional	Triamcinolone acetonide (10–40 mg/mL)	0.1–0.5 mL	Additional injection can be given at 2 weeks for residual lesions
		Sclerosing agents (0.5% sodium tetradecyl sulfate, hypertonic saline, etc.)	0.2–0.3 mL	

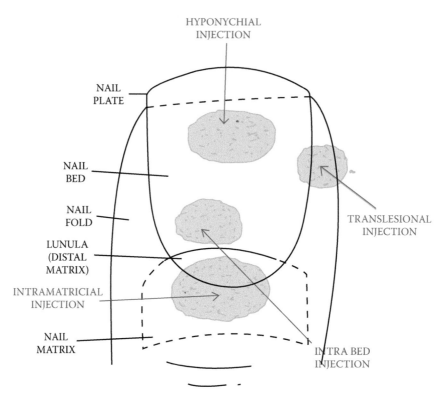

HYPONYCHIAL
INJECTION

NAIL
PLATE

NAIL
BED

NAIL
FOLD

LUNULA
(DISTAL
MATRIX)

INTRAMATRICIAL
INJECTION

NAIL
MATRIX

TRANSLESIONAL
INJECTION

INTRA BED
INJECTION

FIGURE 19.2 Schematic diagram showing various modes of intralesional nail therapies. The yellow area represents the area of diffusion of the drug.

Diseases afflicting the nail lead to impaired cosmesis and a significant negative impact on patients' quality of life and ability to function. However, treating them is a challenge. Due to reasons explained above, nail matrix and bed serve as sanctuary sites due to limited bioavailability of topical as well as systemic drugs. In addition, adverse effects associated with prolonged systemic therapy and potential drug interactions may make systemic therapy unjustifiable in patients with predominant or isolated nail involvement. The slow growth of nails adds to this burden of nail disease. Due to these hurdles, nail diseases are often overlooked and not treated effectively.

Intralesional therapy is a way to overcome these limitations. It is a "targeted form of physician administered, intermittent therapy which is capable of producing a 'depot' effect to maintain bioavailability of the drug at the site of action over longer periods of time." It can effectively bypass the need for systemic administration (thus minimizing first-pass metabolism, drug interactions, and potential systemic side effects) or topical administration (which is highly compromised if special vehicles are not used). This makes it a near ideal and promising therapeutic modality for isolated or predominant nail diseases. Intralesional nail therapy refers to injection of a higher concentration of a drug directly into the nail matrix, nail bed, hyponychium, or translesionally. The localized introduction of a drug into a specific site of the nail apparatus helps in maintaining effective drug levels for a longer period of time, preventing potential treatment relapses. An overview of the major indications in which intralesional therapies have been used in nail is summarized in Table 19.1.

Techniques of Intralesional Nail Therapy

Intralesional injections for nail diseases are easily and efficiently done as an outpatient office procedure. The post-injection period is expected to be uneventful, and the patient can resume normal activities

TABLE 19.2

Individual Nail Manifestations as a Guide to Choose Mode of Intralesional Therapy

Nail manifestation	Probable inflammatory etiology	Site of pathologic involvement	Where to inject?
Nail pitting	Psoriasis, Psoriatic arthritis, Lichen planus, Alopecia areata, Atopic and contact dermatitis	Pits are a result of nail matrix pathology • *Very superficial* pits suggest pathology in the dorsal nail matrix (ventral aspect of proximal nail fold) • *Deeper pits* suggest more extensive involvement of the ventral (germinative nail matrix)	**Nail Matrix** Intramatricial injections
Onychorrhexis	Lichen planus, Nail psoriasis	This also signifies nail matrix pathology. Severity commonly correlates with the degree of effect on matrix	**Nail Matrix** Intramatricial injections
Erythematous lunula	Alopecia areata, Nail psoriasis, Lichen planus, Drug-induced idiopathic *Other causes*: Rheumatoid arthritis, systemic lupus erythematosus, hepatic cirrhosis, carbon monoxide poisoning	Distal matrix	**Nail Matrix** Intramatricial injections
True leukonychia	Nail psoriasis, Nail lichen planus, Idiopathic	Histopathologic correlate is persistence of parakeratotic cells and retained nuclei within the otherwise transparent nail plate. This persistence of parakeratosis is again a sign of proximal matrix pathology	**Nail Matrix** Intramatricial injections
Oil-drop sign or Salmon patch	Nail psoriasis	Nail bed involvement with the disease process	**Nail Bed** Intrabed injections
Distal onychoylsis with subungual hyperkeratosis	Psoriasis, Nail lichen planus, Onychomycosis (no clinical reports of injectable antifungals, only experimental data), Subungual wart or other subungual tumors	Nail bed and Hyponychium	**Nail Bed** Intrabed injections **Hyponychium** Hyponychial injections
Total dystrophic nail (crumbling and destruction)	Nail psoriasis, Nail lichen planus, Total dystrophic onychomycosis (no clinical reports of injectable antifungals, only experimental data)	Nail matrix and nail bed	**Nail Matrix** Intramatricial injections **Nail Bed** Intrabed injections
Space-occupying lesion or tumescent swelling (nail fold)	Myxoid pseudocyst, Subungual/ periungual wart	Nail fold epithelium or underlying structures	**Nail fold** Translesional injection

(a)   (b)

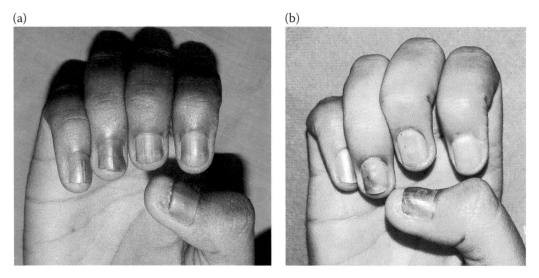

FIGURE 19.3   (a, b) Response to intrabed triamcinolone acetonide in a case of nail psoriasis over 6 months.

(a)   (b)

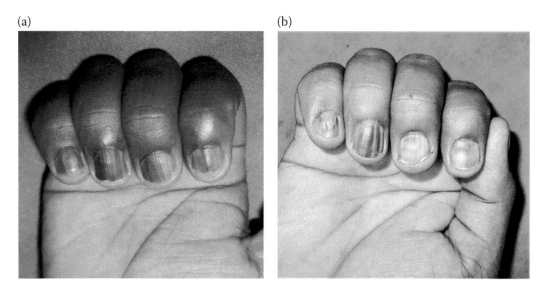

FIGURE 19.4   (a, b) Response to intramatricial triamcinolone acetonide in a case of nail lichen planus.

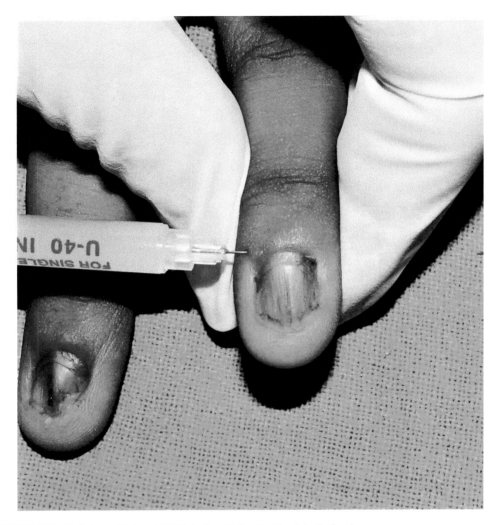

FIGURE 19.5   Technique of intramatricial injection. Notice the blanch in the lunular area.

soon. If digital anesthesia has not been administered (which we normally do not use!), there is no expected downtime, even though a minority of patients can perceive tingling or some numbness till the day end. If digital block has been used, the duration of anesthesia will depend on the anesthetic agent used.

Various techniques are described for reaching specific parts of the nail unit. The part of the nail unit to be treated should be decided based on the predominant nail manifestations. The inflammatory or tumoral nail diseases result in a spectrum of nail manifestations depending on the nail unit area involved with the disease process. Based on this, recognizing the primary area affected within the nail unit helps in deciding the type of injectable therapy to be administered (Figure 19.2) (Table 19.2). Injectable microsphere formulation of terbinafine for drug delivery has been tried in cadaver toe models for potential use in onychomycosis.

Even with an adequate drug delivery, there is a usual lag period before any visible improvement can be seen in the nail changes (Figure 19.3a,b). This is even longer for nail matrix injections and depends on the rate of growth of the treated nail. If a marked or complete improvement is achieved, extending the time interval between injections (once every 6–8 weeks) should be considered. A change of treatment should be considered if there is no clinical response after 3–6 injections.

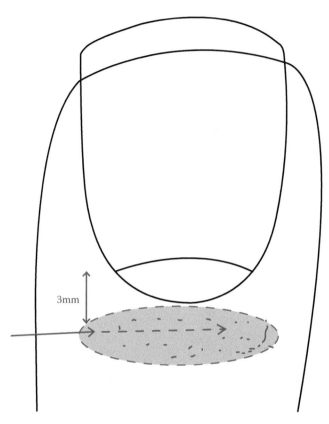

FIGURE 19.6   Gerstein's technique "injecting the drug (0.2-0.25ml) in an even distribution along a line 3mm proximal and parallel to the anterior nail fold at the level of the nail."

All injections in the nail unit should be administered using a 30-gauge needle, preferably a 1-mL Luer-lock syringe or insulin syringe with a built-in needle to minimize pain during needle entry and prevent needle displacement and backsplash. The following are the various techniques of intralesional therapy in nail diseases.

Intramatricial (Nail Matrix) Injection

Intramatricial injection refers to injection of a drug directly into the nail matrix in diseases where the nail matrix is primarily affected. To a small extent, nail bed and nail fold changes are also benefitted with this form of therapy. Toenail disease responds lesser than fingernails to these injections, probably due to the larger size of toe nails, slower rate of nail growth, and higher susceptibility to Koebner's phenomenon from trivial trauma while walking.

The improvement in nail disease achieved with intramatricial therapy can be monitored with the help of validated scoring systems or by using the patient and clinician's 5-point scale of improvement. The score chosen can be recorded at baseline and before every injection during follow-up.

Although the major indications for intramatricial injections over the years have been nail psoriasis and nail lichen planus, other nail diseases are being increasingly treated by this modality include trachyonychia (twenty nail dystrophy) and lichen striatus. There have also been report of nail lichen striatus and trachyonychia responding to intramatricial platelet-rich plasma (PRP) injections. The current nail expert group consensus recommends intramatricial injection of TA as the first line of treatment for isolated classical nail lichen planus (any number of nails) (Figure 19.4a,b) and nail psoriasis involving few nails (≤3 nails involved).

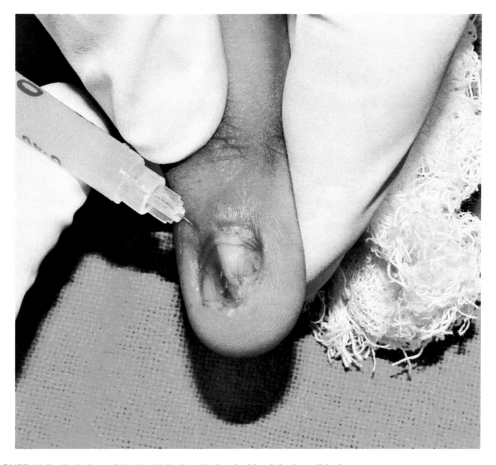

FIGURE 19.7   Technique of intrabed injection. Notice the blanch in the nail bed.

Procedure

Injection into the nail matrix can be placed in various ways, of which technically the easiest would be the Grover technique, where after cleaning the digit with povidone iodine and spirit, the needle is inserted 2 mm below and lateral to the junction between the proximal and the lateral nail folds into the proximal nail matrix, entry into which is indicated by a loss of resistance (Figure 19.5). At times, there is resistance to the penetration of the needle into the nail matrix due to the curvatures of the nail plate. Such a scenario requires slight withdrawal of the needle and reintroduction at a slightly different angle to gain access to the nail matrix. Once in place, the drug is slowly injected to infiltrate the matrix. The endpoint of injection is indicated by a semilunar blanching of the lunula, noticed arising from underneath the proximal nail fold. It indicates the correct site for deposition of the drug (Figure 19.5). After withdrawal of the needle, adequate pressure is applied over the injection site for a minute or so to prevent hematoma formation. Gerstein's technique of intramatricial injection involves "injecting the drug (0.2-0.25ml) in an even distribution along a line 3mm proximal and parallel to the anterior nail fold at the level of the nail." (Figure 19.6). deBerker's technique involves injecting from both sides to deposit the drug in the nail matrix area.

Intrabed (Nail Bed) Injection

In this technique, the drug is deposited directly into the nail bed for diseases producing changes predominantly in the nail bed like distal onycholysis, salmon patch, pustules, or subungual hyperkeratosis. As the nail bed is a tightly contained space because of the overlying unyielding nail plate, drug

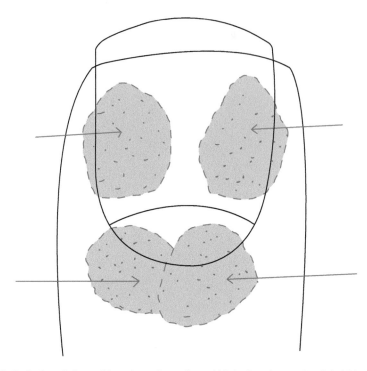

FIGURE 19.8 DeBerker's technique of four site periungual steroid injection given under digital block.

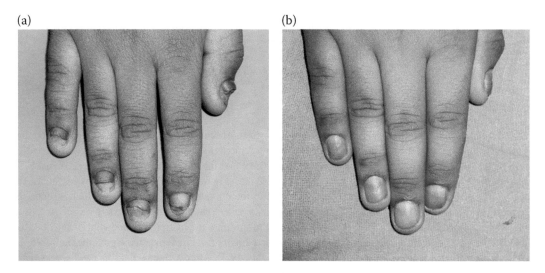

FIGURE 19.9 (a, b) Response to nail bed steroid injections in a patient with nail psoriasis.

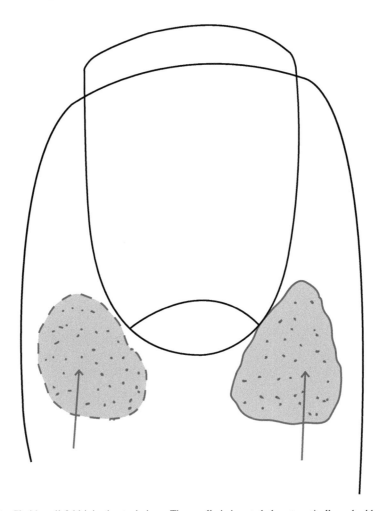

FIGURE 19.10 Clark's nail fold injection technique. The needle is inserted almost vertically and a blanch is noticed in the periungual tissue. Slow diffusion of the drug occurs thereafter.

deposition is more painful due to the pressure produced against nerve fibers. TA and methotrexate are the drugs which have been used with this technique for treating nail psoriasis, the dosage and interval maybe kept similar to intramatricial injection.

Procedure

As nail bed injection is more painful compared to nail matrix injections, it may be performed under local anesthesia (either infiltrative or nerve block), especially for the uninitiated or if multiple injections are required. Different approaches have been suggested for drug deposition into nail bed like direct penetration of the nail plate, injection via the hyponychium, injection via the lateral nail fold (directing the needle medially towards the nail bed), and injection via the proximal nail fold. Injection via the proximal nail fold (Grover 2017a) is preferred in view of minimal procedural pain obviating the need for digital anesthesia (Figure 19.7). After patient preparation and proper positioning, the needle is inserted in a plane similar to the nail matrix injection. However, the point of insertion in the proximal nail fold is more medial as compared to intramatricial injection. The needle is advanced medially and distally towards the center of the nail to penetrate the nail bed (Figure 19.7). The drug is then injected slowly till no more can enter. The end-point is seen as a blanching effect of the nail bed with the blanch arising

(a)   (b)

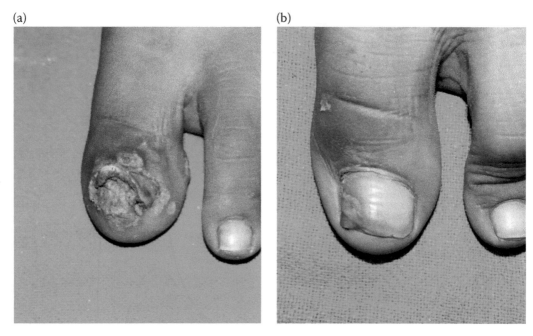

FIGURE 19.11   Response to bleomycin injections in a case of distally placed subungual and periungual warts.

more distally as compared to the intramatricial injection (Figure 19.7). The needle is then slowly withdrawn ensuring adequate hemostasis. In the deBerker technique, 0.1 mL of TA is injected in each of the four quadrants of the nail unit per session approaching from the lateral nail fold, targeting nail matrix disease along with nail bed disease in nail psoriasis after standard proximal ring block (Figure 19.8). This technique showed maximum benefit in subungual hyperkeratosis (nail bed disease) and least benefit in pitting (nail matrix disease). Nail bed injections give acceptable results in patients with nail bed psoriasis (Figure 19.9a,b).

Intrafold Injection

In this technique, injections are given into the nail fold dermis with the drug diffusing into the nail matrix and proximal nail bed, thereby avoiding painful injections into nail matrix or bed. This technique works on the principle that the nail matrix epithelium has more dermis overlying it in the nail fold than beneath it, thereby acting as a depot place from where the drug can slowly diffuse (Figure 19.10). This method is useful for diseases predominantly affecting the proximal nail fold and nail matrix like chronic paronychia, nail changes associated with hand eczema, nail lichen planus, trachyonychia, and some cases of nail psoriasis. It is not much effective in treating distal nail bed/hyponychial disease. It was seen that nail pitting responds better to injection into the nail fold than into the nail matrix, illustrating a role of the proximal nail fold in the pathogenesis of pits. Hoigné syndrome is a side effect reported with triamicinolone injection via this technique.

Hyponychial Injection

In this technique, the distal nail bed is approached via the hyponychium. It is useful for distal nail bed changes like distal onycholysis and subungual hyperkeratosis in psoriasis, distal subungual warts (Figure 19.11a,b); or for very large nails (e.g., nails of great toe), where the drug injected into nail matrix or bed might not be sufficient enough to diffuse into the most distal parts of the nail (Figure 19.12). Prior digital anesthesia is mostly required as pain is expectedly higher due to needle entry through a more sensitive part of the nail unit. In the Richert technique, injections are placed in

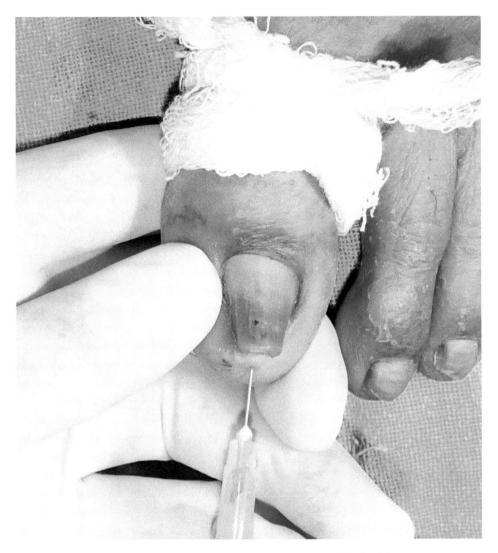

FIGURE 19.12   Technique of hyponychial injection in a case of nail psoriasis with distal changes.

each of the four quadrants of the nail in a fan-shaped manner under the nail plate through the hypo-nychium for the treatment of nail psoriasis.

Translesional Injection

In case of a space-occupying lesions involving the nail unit, an injection into the substance of the lesion is required (translesional injection) (Figure 19.13). A number of drugs with varied mechanism of action can be used via this technique, for the management of nail unit tumors like periungual or subungual warts, or myxoid pseudocysts involving the proximal nail fold. Intralesional bleomycin is a very effective modality for the treatment of periungual and subungual warts as the concentration of bleomycin hydrolase that inactivates bleomycin is very minimal in the nail unit. It is useful in warts which are recalcitrant to other forms of destructive therapy, with an added benefit of being effective even in

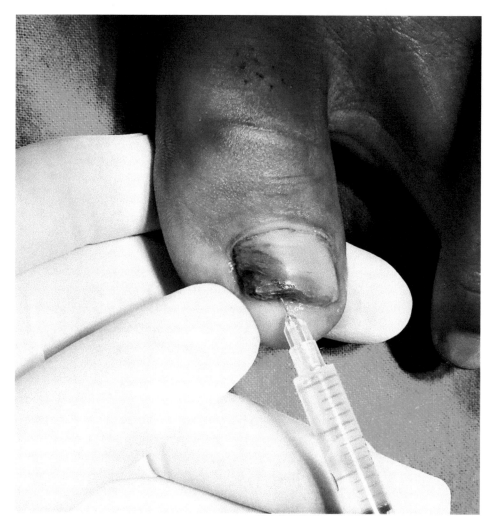

FIGURE 19.13 Technique of translesional injection in a subungual wart.

immunocompromised patients unlike the other injectable forms of immunotherapy. Various immunotherapeutic modalities used in the nail unit warts include intralesional MMR (Measles, Mumps,
Rubella) vaccine, Mw (Mycobacterium w) vaccine, and Vitamin D injection. They offer the advantage
of clearance of warts at sites distant from the site of injection.

Procedure

Translesional injection of bleomycin in periungual or subungual warts can be administered by various
techniques.

- Direct infiltration into the wart tissue using a Luer-lock syringe or insulin syringe and is the
  preferred technique for subungual warts (Figure 19.13). Care must be taken by the provider to
  protect the eyes (wear protective eye shield or face shield) as the injected drug can backsplash

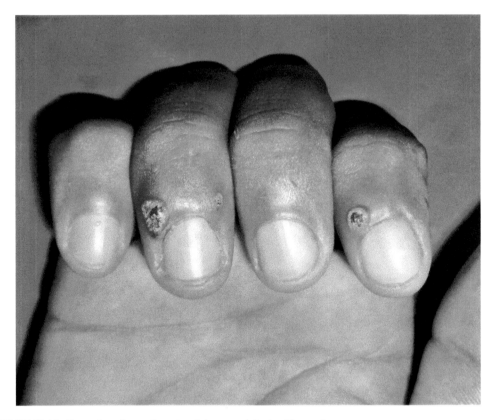

FIGURE 19.14 Formation of necrotic eschar 2 days post injection bleomycin.

due to the dry and fissured surface of the warts. This is the only method which can target even subungual warts without having to remove the overlying nail plate.

- In Shelley and Shelley technique of bleopuncture, a drop of bleomycin is applied on the surface of the wart and keeping the skin taut, multiple punctures are made using a bifurcated vaccination needle or an insulin syringe to penetrate the wart (40 times/5 mm^2). This is followed by application of a dry dressing. This method is also useful in the treatment of palmoplantar warts.
- Microneedling with topical spray of bleomycin solution followed by occlusion can be done to allow the drug to percolate into the wart tissue. As can be seen, both the latter methods are useful for periungual spread of the wart, but not so much for the subungual extensions.

Prior to bleopuncture, the digit can be soaked in water to hydrate the wart keratin so as to facilitate the process and reduce the resistance encountered. For bleomycin, the injection must be placed into each and every wart for complete treatment. The endpoint while injecting bleomycin is a blanching or yellowish appearance of the wart due to vasoconstriction. One can even see small microdroplets of the solution exuding over the surface once signaling that the wart has been completely infiltrated. Post procedure, a necrotic eschar (with occasional bulla formation) develops on the treated areas over the next 2–3 days (Figure 19.14). This is followed by shrinkage and shedding of wart tissue in the form of a

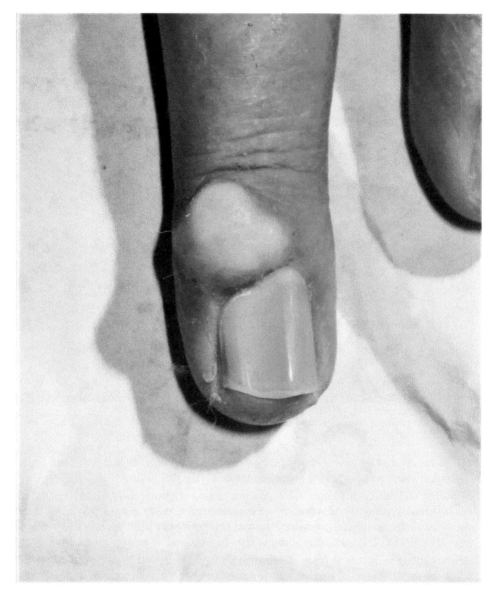

FIGURE 19.15 Technique of translesional injection in a myxoid cyst. Note the blanch and swelling produced post injection.

brown keratotic scale overlying smooth skin without bleeding points over the next 1–2 weeks. The patient is advised to apply liberal quantities of emollients over the treated warts to prevent fissuring and pain while the eschar forms and sheds. For immunotherapy with Vitamin D, MMR and Mw vaccine, the injection is infiltrated directly into the wart tissue in one or two of the largest warts only.

In the case of myxoid pseudocyst, the drug (TA or sclerosant) is injected directly into the cyst cavity after evacuation of the mucinous material (Figure 19.15). The endpoint is a blanch and a turgidity of the

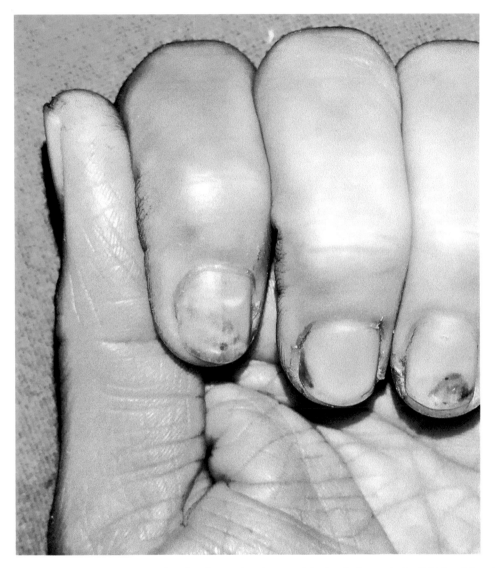

FIGURE 19.16   Blackish spots seen at the point of entry of methotrexate injection (in the proximal nail fold) and the point of drug deposition (in the nail bed).

pseudocyst, which indicates correct filling of the lesion. This is followed by immediate compression dressing with an elastic bandage for 24 hours. This technique is useful for smaller lesions, or to reduce the size of larger lesions before attempting surgical intervention.

Needle-Free Intradermal Injection

Jet injection is defined as a needle-free drug delivery system, which utilizes a high-speed stream of fluid containing the drug to penetrate the skin and deposit in the dermis. Needle-free intradermal injection

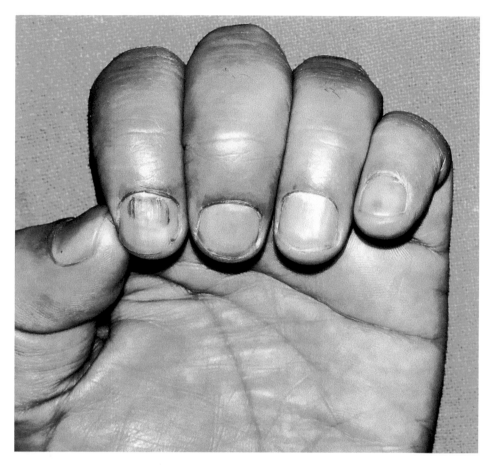

FIGURE 19.17   Subungual hematoma formation after the previous injection 4 weeks prior.

(NFII) can be of two types: spring-loaded jet injector (Dermojet/Port-O-Jet) and gas-powered jet injector. Needleless injectors not only reduce the pain during drug delivery but also confine the drug more evenly in the dermis at the desired penetration level. However, they have inherent disadvantages like clogging of the injector, backsplash, and risk of spread of blood-borne infection (because of difficulty in sterilizing the apparatus). There have also been reports of multiple implantation epidermoid cysts formation following treatment of psoriatic nails requiring amputation. These have been used in intramatricial drug delivery for nail psoriasis and can also be used for drug delivery in other nail diseases. With the advent of disposable jet injectors/cartridges, autoclaving of the injector remains the only reliable method to eliminate the risk of infection.

Limited literature is available regarding injectable therapy in acquired nail dystrophies like nail psoriasis, nail lichen planus, or trachyonychia, and ungual warts. The studies suffer from varying treatment protocols, assessment tools, and duration of follow-up. Table 19.3 summarizes these studies.

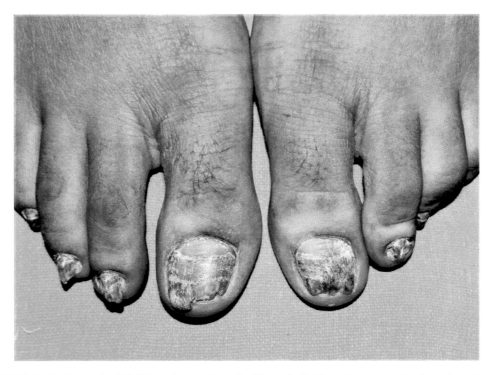

FIGURE 19.18 Proximal nail fold hypopigmentation and mild atrophy in bilateral great toe nails of a patient with nail psoriasis. The nail is partially improved.

Pre-Treatment Considerations

For any form of intralesional nail therapy, an informed written consent should be taken as this is an invasive approach. The patient should surely be explained the need for treatment, other treatment options available, and the advantages and disadvantages of injectables vis-à-vis other forms of therapy. For consenting patients, a pre-procedure (baseline) photographic documentation should also be done, showing all involved nails clearly. This is because treatment results are slow to appear and may be incomplete in many cases. Ideally, photograph in same position and lighting should be taken before each injection administration. While treating with drugs like methotrexate and cyclosporine, baseline complete blood counts, and liver function tests can be performed; however, there is no consensus on the need for such blood investigations at baseline or at successive injections. One should also rule out the absolute and relative contraindications to intralesional nail therapies before initiating the procedure (Table 19.4).

For the procedure, we make the patient lie down in a prone position with the hand extended toward the operator. This gives best access for the nail unit at different angles. It also minimizes the risk of vasovagal syncopal attack due to the perceived pain of needle entry.

Pain during injection is one of the major drawbacks of this form of therapy and one of the major causes for patients and/or providers not choosing this form of therapy. It is also a cause of low patient compliance and treatment drop-out. However, procedure-related pain can be minimized by few simple techniques which are listed in Table 19.5.

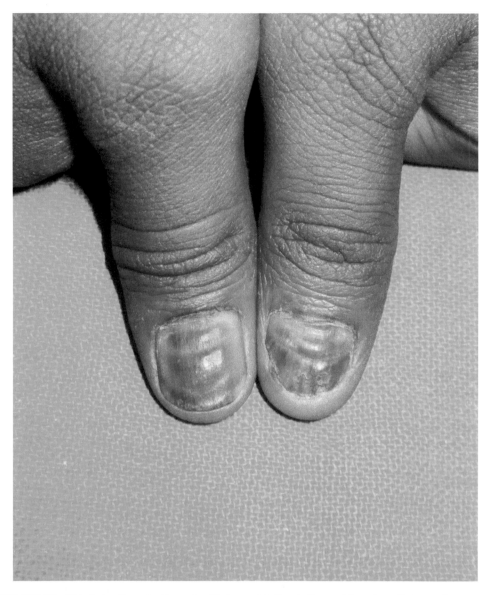

FIGURE 19.19   Disturbed pattern of nail growth with incomplete Beau's lines and irregular nail plate surface.

Adverse Effects of Intralesional Nail Therapies

Though the treatment is generally considered safe, intralesional nail therapy, like any other form of therapy, is not devoid of side effects. These can range from mostly trivial effects, which can be minimized by careful technique, to the severe ones rarely including gangrenous changes and systemic drug diffusion. The side effects reported in literature are summarized in Table 19.6. However, these can be avoided if the drug is injected using the appropriate technique and the correct dosing.

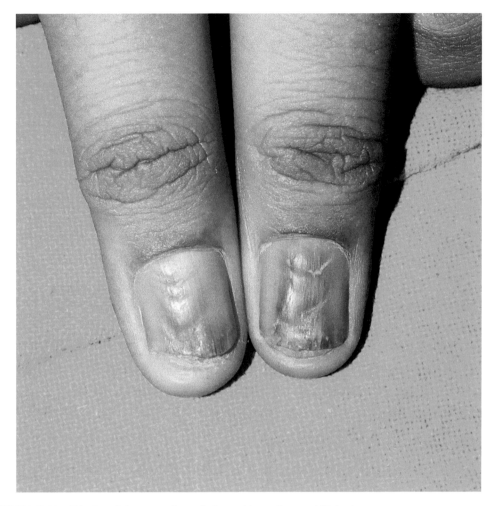

FIGURE 19.20 Thinning of the outgrowing nail plates with ongoing steroid injections.

It is possible that a larger particle size of drug injected may incite vascular occlusion phenomena. Baran (2014) described a case of Hoigné syndrome, wherein a patient given triamcinolone acetonide in the proximal nail fold developed dorsal pain, dyspnea, and headache immediately post injection. Grover et al. (2017b) described another case where a young male with nail lichen planus, developed Nicolau syndrome (extensive ischemic necrosis and gangrenous changes surrounding the site of intramatricial injection site). Fortunately, both these side effects are very rare and were reversible.

Summary

Intralesional nail therapy is a promising form of drug delivery in nail disorders. It is especially useful in patients with isolated nail involvement to avoid side effects associated with systemic forms of therapy. Proper selection of patients and the technique to be followed helps achieve optimal results. Having said

TABLE 19.3

Summary of Studies on Intralesional Therapies in Common Nail Diseases

Authors, year	Indication	Site	Agent used	No. of patients	Results
Gerstein, 1962	Nail psoriasis	Nail matrix	TA (10 mg/mL, 0.2–0.25 mL)	4 patients (15 nails)	Variable response lasting for 6 months
DeBerker & Lawrence, 1998		Nail matrix and nail bed	TA (10 mg/mL, 0.4 mL) at 3-monthly intervals	19 patients (46 nails)	Subungual hyperkeratosis and nail thickening showed maximum benefit
Grover et al., 2005		Nail matrix	TA (5 mg/mL, 0.1–0.2 mL) 4 weekly × 6 months	4 patients	One patient showed 75–100% improvement
Grover et al., 2017		Nail bed	Methotrexate (25 mg/mL, 0.1 mL) 3 weekly × 5 sessions	4 patients (30 nails)	Decline in mean NAPSI from 4.87 to 2.17
Mittal & Mahajan, 2018		Nail matrix	TA (10 mg/mL, 0.1 mL) MTX (25 mg/mL, 0.1 mL) CyA (50 mg/mL, 0.1 mL)30 nails each; Repeat injection at 6 weeks	17 patients (90 fingernails)	>75% improvement in 50% nails in TA and Methotrexate group, and 33% in cyclosporine group
Grover et al., 2005	Nail lichen planus	Nail matrix	TA (5 mg/mL, 0.1–0.2 mL) at monthly intervals × 6 months	12 patients	One-third patients showed 75–100% response
Piraccini et al., 2010		Nail matrix	TA (10 mg/mL, 0.4 mL) at monthly intervals	8 patients	7/8 patients showed complete regression of nail symptoms after 4–7 injections
Khoo et al., 2000	Trachyonychia	Nail matrix	TA (10 mg/mL, 0.05 mL) 8 weekly × 3 sessions	4 patients (all patients are <12 years old)	Pitting decreased to mean of 15% at 2 months, increased to 42% at 4 months
Grover et al., 2005		Nail matrix	TA (5 mg/mL, 0.1–0.2 mL) 4 weekly × 6 months	34 patients	11 patients showed 75–100% improvement
Yoo et al., 2020	Nail dystrophy (psoriasis, lichen planus, trauma, hand eczema)	Nail matrix and proximal nail fold	TA (2.5 mg/mL, 0.1 mL) 4 weekly × 6–12 months	12 patients (55 nails)	3 and 5 patients had 75–100% and 50–75% improvement, respectively
Shelley & Shelley, 1991	Mutiple sites including periungual warts	Puncture with bifurcated needle	Bleomycin (1 U/mL, 0.02 mL/5 mm^2 onto wart surface)	66 patients (258 warts)	92% warts cleared completely regardless of the site

(Continued)

TABLE 19.3 (*Continued*)

Authors, year	Indication	Site	Agent used	No. of patients	Results
Soni et al., 2011	Periungual wart	Intralesional injection	Bleomycin (1 U/mL, 0.2–1 mL, depending on size of wart), repeated at 2 weeks if needed	5 patients (8 warts)	Complete resolution of lesions after 1 or 2 injections
Alghamdi and Khurram; 2011		Translesional multipuncture technique	Bleomycin (1 U/mL, 0.3–0.6 mL) every 4 weeks	15 patients (15 warts treated)	86.6% had complete clearance, 50% patients with multiple warts had clearance of untreated lesions

Note: TA: Triamcinolone acetonide; MTX: Methotrexate; CyA: Cyclosporine A.

TABLE 19.4

Contraindications for Intralesional Therapy

Absolute

- Known hypersensitivity to the drug used

Relative

- Active infection at the injection site
- Bleeding diathesis
- Peripheral vascular disease
- Raynaud's phenomenon
- Uncontrolled diabetes or hypertension
- Unrealistic expectations of the patient
- Too young and uncooperative patients

that, nail diseases can be refractory to injectables at times, and different features may respond variably to different techniques. One should be aware of the immediate and delayed complications possible, to prevent and treat them at the earliest. Injectables are still an infrequently performed procedure in routine nail practice and is a field yet to be explored further.

- The choice of type of injectable therapy should be guided by the clinical features of the nail unit.
- Common indications of injectable, therapy, include isolated nail involvement in psoriasis and lichen planus, trachyonychia, and subungual and periungual warts.
- The dermatologist should be aware of the techniques to minimize patient discomfort while injecting which can be done without digital anesthesia.

TABLE 19.5

Ways to Minimize Pain during Intralesional Nail Therapies

Prior to injection	
	1. Use of topical anesthesia (EMLA under occlusion) for 1 hour
	2. Use of icepacks/cold air/vibration/pressure on the digit prior to injection can decrease the entry pain of the needle
	3. Treatment can be given under digital block to the most apprehensive patients (if treatment planned for few nails)
	4. Injectable solution should be at body temperature at the time of use to prevent the initial stinging sensation
During injection	
	1. Injection should be placed using the thinnest needles (e.g., 30-G needle) with the bevel side up
	2. The entry point of injection should be through the relatively thinner skinned dorsal aspect of finger
	3. Verbal reassurances and conversation while injecting (talkesthesia) helps
	4. Injection should be given slowly as drug infusion is more painful (due to the confined tissue space) than needle entry
	5. Needle-free jet injectors can minimize pain with added advantage of delivering the injection at the desired penetration level

TABLE 19.6

Side Effects of Intralesional Nail Therapies

Side effects of intramatricial/intrabed injections	Side effects of translesional injection
Local	*Due to bleomycin*
Common	**Common**
Injection site pain (may last for minutes to days, maximum with cyclosporine)	Injection site pain (may last for up to 24 hours)
Transient post injection numbness	Erythema and edema at the site of injection (may last up to 72 hours)
Blackish discoloration (with methotrexate injection) (Figure 19.16)	
	Uncommon
Uncommon	Severe pain
Subungual hematoma (Figure 19.17)	Ulceration at the site of injection
Traumatic leukonychia	Raynaud's phenomena
Proximal nail fold hypopigmentation and/or atrophy (Figure 19.18) (with TA if used at too high dosage, too superficial, too frequent, or for too long)	Fingertip gangrene
	Onychomades is
	Scarring and permanent onychodystrophy
Disturbed nail growth (Figure 19.19)	*Due to immunotherapy*
Proximal onycholysis	**Common**
Thinning of nail plate (with TA) (Figure 19.20)	Injection site pain
Splitting and distortion of the nail plate (seen with methotrexate and cyclosporine)	**Uncommon**
Acute paronychia (with TA)	High-grade fever
	Redness and/ or swelling Induration and ulcer formation at the injection site
Rare	*Following treatment of myxoid pseudocyst*
Disappearance of the phalanx under injection	**Common**
Tendon rupture (with TA)	Local pain
Nicolau syndrome (in case of nail matrix injection in lichen planus)	Erythema and/or edema
	Nail fold atrophy/hypopigmentation (with TA)
Systemic	**Uncommon**
Hoigne syndrome	Ulceration and/or necrosis.
Vasovagal attack	
Hypersensitivity reactions	

BIBLIOGRAPHY

Abell A., Samman PD (1973) Intradermal triamcinolone treatment of nail dystrophies. *Br J Dermatol*; 89: 191–197.

AlGhamdi K. M., Khurram H. (2011) Successful treatment of periungual warts with diluted bleomycin using translesional multipuncture technique: A pilot prospective study. *Dermatol Surg*; 37: 486–492.

Al-Naggar M. R., Al-Adl A.S., Rabie A. R., Abdelkhalk M. R., Elsaie M.L. (2019) Intralesional bleomycin injection vs microneedling-assisted topical bleomycin spraying in treatment of plantar warts. *J Cosmet Dermatol*; 18(1): 124–128.

Angamuthu Nanjappa S. H., Raman V. (2014) Controlled-release injectable containing Terbinafine/PLGA microspheres for Onychomycosis Treatment. *J Pharma Sci*; 103: 1178–1183.

Awal G., Kaur S. (2018) Therapeutic outcome of intralesional immunotherapy in cutaneous warts using the Mumps, Measles, and Rubella vaccine: A randomized, placebo-controlled Trial. *J Clin Aesthet Dermatol*; 11: 15–20.

Baran R. (2014) Proximal nail fold intralesional steroid injection responsible for Hoigné syndrome. *JEADV*; 11: 1563–1565 (online Oct 2013).

Brauns B., Stahl M., Schon M. P., Zutt M. (2011) Intralesional steroid injection alleviates nail lichen planus. *Int Ju Dermatol*; 50: 626–627.

Clark A., Jellinek N. J. (2016) Intralesional injection for inflammatory nail diseases. *Dermatol Surg*; 42(2): 257–260.

DeBerker D.A., Lawrence C. M. (1998) A simplified protocol of steroid injection for psoriatic nail dystrophy. *Br J Dermatol*; 138(1): 90–95.

Garg S., Baveja S. (2014) Intralesional immunotherapy for difficult to treat warts with Mycobacterium w vaccine. *J Cutan Aesthet Surg*; 7(4): 203–208.

Gerstein W. (1962) Psoriasis and lichen planus of nails. *Treatment with triamcinolone. Arch Dermatol*; 86: 419–421.

Grover C., Bansal S. (2018) A compendium of intralesional therapies in nail disorders. *Indian Dermatol Online J*; 9: 373–382.

Grover C., Bansal S., Nanda S., Reddy B. S. (2005) Efficacy of triamcinolone acetonide in various acquired nail dystrophies. *J Dermatol*; 32(12): 963–968.

Grover C., Kharghoria G., Daulatabad D., Bhattacharya S. N. (2017) Nicolau syndrome following intramatricial triamcinolone injection for nail lichen planus. *Indian Dermatol Online J*; 8(5): 350–351.

Grover C., Daulatabad D., Singal A. (2017) Role of nail bed methotrexate injections in isolated nail psoriasis: conventional drug via an unconventional route. *Clin Exp Dermatol*; 42(4): 420–423.

Gupta M. K., Geizhals S., Lipner S. R. (2019) Intralesional triamcinolone matrix injections for treatment of trachyonychia. *J Am Acad Dermatol*; S0190-9622(19): 32809–32809.

Iorizzo M., Tosti A., Starace M., et al. (2020) Isolated nail lichen planus: an expert consensus on treatment of the classical form. *J Am Acad Dermatol*; S0190-9622(20): 30300–30305.

Jakhar D., Kaur I., Misri R. (2019) Intralesional vitamin D3 in periungual warts. *J Am Acad Dermatol*; 80(5): e111–e112.

Kaur I., Jakhar D. (2019) Intramatricial platelet-rich plasma therapy: a novel treatment modality in refractory nail disorders. *Dermatol Ther*; 32(2): e12831.

Kavya M., Shashikumar B. M., Harish M. R., Shweta B. P. (2017) Safety and efficacy of intralesional vitamin D3 in cutaneous warts: an open uncontrolled trial. *J Cutan Aesthet Surg*; 10(2): 90–94.

Kerure A. S., Nath A. K., Oudeacoumar P. (2016) Intralesional immunotherapy with tuberculin purified protein derivative for verruca: a study from a teaching hospital in South India. *Indian J Dermatol Venereol Leprol*; 82: 420–422.

Khoo B. P., Giam Y.C. (2000) A pilot study on the role of intralesional triamcinolone acetonide in the treatment of pitted nails in children. *Singapore Med J*; 41: 66–68.

Lewis T. G., Nydorf E. D. (2006) Intralesional bleomycin for wart: a review. *J Drugs Dermatol*; 5: 499–504.

Mittal J., Mahajan B. B. (2018) Intramatricial injections for nail psoriasis: an open-label comparative study of triamcinolone, methotrexate, and cyclosporine. *Indian J Dermatol Venereol Leprol*; 84: 419–423.

Nantel-Battista M., Richer V., Marcil I., Benohanian A. (2014) Treatment of nail psoriasis with intralesional triamcinolone acetonide using a needle-free jet injector: a prospective trial. *J Cutan Med Surg*; 18: 38–42.

Park S. E., Park E. J., Kim S. S., Kim C. W. (2014) Treatment of digital mucous cysts with intralesional sodium tetradecylsulfate injection. *Dermatol Surg*; 40: 1249–1254.

Piraccini B. M., Saccani E., Starace M., Balestri R., Tosti A. (2010) Nail lichen planus: response to treatment and long term follow-up. *Eur J Dermatol*; 20: 489–496.

Rigopoulos D., Baran R., Chiheb S. et al. (2019) Recommendations for the definition, evaluation, and treatment of nail psoriasis in adult patients with no or mild skin psoriasis: a dermatologist and nail expert group consensus. *J Am Acad Dermatol*; 81: 228– 240.

Shelley W. B., Shelley E. D. (1991) Intralesional bleomycin sulfate therapy for warts: A novel bifurcated needle puncture technique. *Arch Dermatol*; 127: 234–236.

Soni P., Khandelwal K., Aara N., Ghiya B. C., Mehta R. D., Bumb R. A. (2011 Sep) Efficacy of Intralesional Bleomycin in Palmo-plantar and Periungual Warts. *J Cutan Aesthet Surg*; 4(3): 188–191.

Yoo K. H., Bang D. S., Han H. S., Li K., Kim B. J. (2020) Intralesional triamcinolone injections for the treatment of nail dystrophy: A case series. *Dermatologic Therapy*; 33: e13427. https://doi.org/10.1111/dth.13427.

20

Drug side effects on the distal phalanx

Robert Baran

Pyogenic granulomas (PGs) are benign vascular lesions that can result from a large number of etio-logical factors, consequently, any drug with angiogenic side effects can cause these tumors.

PGs can be treated through surgery, cryotherapy, cautery, sclerotherapy, or lasers

Recently the use of propranolol cream 1% or timolol gel 0.5 applied on paronychia and/or PGs overnight under occlusion (a plastic wrap) for a maximum of 45 days was reported to be effective. Unfortunately, propranolol did not influence the course of PGs in the toenails in patients (Piraccini et al. 2016) (Figures 20.1 and 20.2).

In addition, there are case-series showing the efficacy of 5-aminolaevulinic acid photodynamic therapy for epidermal growth factor receptor inhibitor-induced paronychia and/or PGs (Panariello et al. 2019).

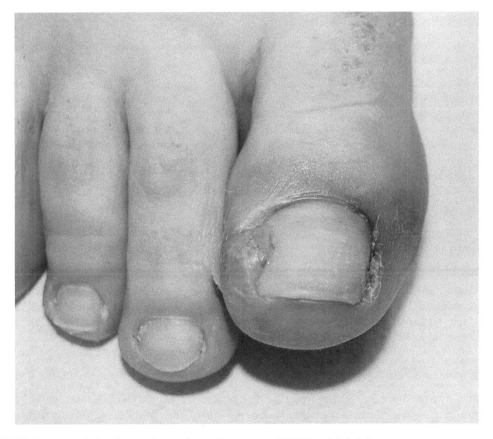

FIGURE 20.1   Drug-induced pyogenic granuloma. (By courtesy of BM Piraccini, Italy.)

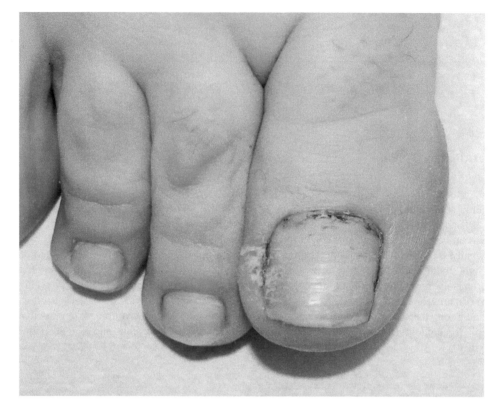

FIGURE 20.2 Same patient as in Figure 20.1, after topical Timolol application under overnight occlusion. (By courtesy of BM Piraccini, Italy.)

Paronychia and periungual pyogenic granulomas represent one of the most common and bothersome dermatologic toxicities observed with ErbB inhibitors. With the use of topical propanolol or of timolol, nearly two-thirds of patients showed at least a partial response after 1 month of therapy (Sibaud et al. 2019).

Topical betaxolol 0.25% eye drops have also been applied once daily for treating relapsing pyogenic granuloma-like lesions induced by epidermal growth factor receptor inhibitors (Yen et al. 2018).

Old and new drugs, may produce side effects now properly treated with old or new topical drugs.

Paronychia and/or Periungual Granuloma

The development of periungual pyogenic granuloma while taking the oral acne drug isotretinoin is a known yet uncommon and potentially serious side effect of the oral vitamin A derivative (Benedetto et al. 2019).

Multiple subungual pyogenic granulomas followed levothyroxine treatment (Keles et al. 2015).

See also Table 20.1.

Paronychia and Periungual Granulation as a Novel Side Effect of Ibrutinib: A Case Report

Ibrutinib, a targeted therapy, is effective in the treatment of chronic lymphocytic leukemia and B-cell malignancies. Brittle are the most commonly reported nail-related side effect. Paronychial inflammation and periungual granulation have been recently described. The patient, a 40-year-old woman, was prescribed boric acid soak and topical corticosteroids; however, she was lost to follow-up (Yorulmaz and Yalcin 2020).

TABLE 20.1

Drug-Induced Pyogenic Granulomas

Acitretin	Indinavir
Anti-TNF-α therapy	Lamivudine
Capecitabine	Levothyroxine
Carbamazepine	mTOR inhibitors
Cetuximab	Retinoids
Docetaxel	Rituximab
Erb B inhibitors Risperidone	Vemurafenib
Gefitinib	Zidovudine
Imatinib	5-Fluorouracil

Paronychia Associated with Ledipasvir/Sofosbuvir for Hepatitis C Treatment

Paronychia involved multiple toenails in a patient undergoing Hepatitis C therapy with L/S. The patient was treated conservatively with topical mupirocin in the morning, clobetasol ointment in the evening, and acetic acid soaks twice daily, resulting in symptomatic improvement and control. However, complete symptom resolution occurred only after completion of his ledipasvir/sofosbuvir treatment (Sampson and Lewis 2019).

Multiple Eruptive Periungual Granuloma during Risperidone Therapy for Schizophrenia

A 26-year-old man with schizophrenia presented with a 2 month history of multiple friable papules on the lateral nail folds of fingers and toes. He was receiving a dopaminergic antipsychotic agent, risperidone for 4 months. Topical phenol applications seemed to be a simple and effective treatment for multiple periungual pyogenic granulomas (Zaraa et al. 2013).

Recalcitrant Trametinib-Induced Paronychia Treated Successfully with Topical Timolol in a Drug-Induced Pediatric Patient

Paronychia has been described as a side effect in patients undergoing treatment with MED (mitogen-activated protein kinase enzyme) inhibitors. It is usually a recurrent condition that can have a significant impact on the quality of life. Topical beta-blocker treatment has been described as an effective therapy in antineoplastic drug induced pyogenic granuloma and in antineoplastic drug induced paronychia. The authors described the first case treated with timolol gel 0.5% for a trametinib-induced paronychia in a pediatric patient that allowed to continue the third line antineoplastic therapy for his glioma (Martinez de Espronceda et al. 2020).

Tenofovir Disoproxil Fumarate used for chronic hepatitis B may be responsible of nail pitting (Sari 2018).

Median Nail Dystrophy

This uncommon idiopathic dystrophy typically appears as central longitudinal groove or split involving one or both thumbnails. Unusual longitudinal thumb fissures were caused by **Erlotinib** therapy for metastatic lung cancer (Desanu et al. 2018).

A 53-year-old man presented with median canaliform nail dystrophy treated with **1064-nm quasi long-pulsed Nd:YAG laser** (Choi et al. 2017).

Ritonavir associated with **Lopinavir** inhibits HIV protease and may produce a median nail dystrophy of the thumbs (Borges-Costa and Sacramento Marques 2013).

Isotretinoin may be responsible for the same disorder (Dharmagunawardena and Charles-Holmès 1997).

Angiotensin-Convertine Inhibitors and Lichen Planus

Irbesartan used to lower blood pressure of a 77-year-old patient was responsible for pain of the nail unit involving all digits 6 months after beginning of her treatment. This symptom was associated with progressive nail dystrophy leading to the clinical diagnosis of lichen planus that was confirmed histologically (Bories and Denis 2005).

Voriconazole therapy was associated with nail changes in 106 patients (70%) out of 152, including nail loss in 15, split nail in 20, thinning of the nails in 16 (Borges-Costa and Sacramento Marques 2013).

Teriflunomide has been reported to induce psoriasiform changes of fingernails: It is the active metabolite of leflunomide, currently used as an immunomodulatory agent in multiple sclerosis. The authors report the rapid onset of psoriasiform changes on fingernails induced by this molecule in multiple sclerosis, which raises the issue of a paradoxical reactions reminiscent of those observed with anti-TNF alpha agents when used in nondermatological indications (Dereure and Camu 2017). **Nail loss after teriflunomide treatment** is a new potential adverse event (Mancinelli et al. 2017).

Lichenoid drug eruption with antituberculosis drugs (rifampicin and izoniazid) was associated with a permanent anonychia and dorsal pterygium is a rare condition (BayBay 2020).

Disappearing Digit Due to Topical Corticosteroids

This condition was named by tanenbaum as topical steroid atrophy *"a disappearing digit,"* then *"distal phalangeal atrophy secondary to topical steroid therapy"* by Deffer and Goette, and finally *"corticosteroid-induced disappearing digit"* by Wolf et al. (1990).

Usually the patients present with large erythemato-squamous distal fingers and a marked shortening of the nail beds. Sometimes there is a sclerodermiform appearance of the dorsal digits, a shortening of the nail plates and disappearance of the lunula caused by a distal extension of the proximal nail fold (Figure 20.3).

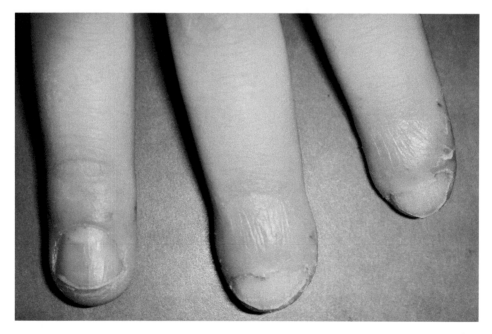

FIGURE 20.3   Corticosteroid-induced disappearing digit with shortening of the phalanx. (By courtesy of J. André, Belgium.)

This side effect secondary to topical steroid therapy may even present with a subtotal disappearance of the phalangeal bones in elderly (Degreef and de Smet 2007).

Beneficial Drug Effects

Topical 20% sodium thiosulfate was applied three times a day on calcinosis cutis of fingertip in CREST syndrome with success after 3 years (Tajalli and Qureschi 2019).

5% Topical minoxidil solution was applied twice-daily to the fingernails of 32 participants. During the first month, the mean growth of the treated nails was 4.27 mm/month compared with 3.91 mm/month in the untreated nails (*P* 0.003). These findings suggest that a 5% concentration of topical minoxidil can stimulate nail growth with increased growth beginning in the first week of application (Mempanakit et al. 2017).

BIBLIOGRAPHY

BayBay H., Saâdani C., Elloudi S. et al. (2020) Lichenoïd drug eruption with antituberculosis drugs associated with an anonychia. *Ann Dermatol Venereol*; 147: 456–460.

Benedetto C., Crasto D., Ettefagh L. et al. (2019) Development of periungual pyogenic granuloma with associated paronychia following isotretinoin therapy. A case report and a review of the literature. *J Clin Aesthet Dermatol*; 12: 32–36.

Borges-Costa J., Sacramento Marques M. (2013) Median nail dystrophy associated with Ritonavir. *Int J Dermatol*; 52: 1581–1582.

Bories A., Denis P. (2005) Dystrophie unguéale lichénoïde induite par les inhibiteurs de l'angiotensine 2. *Ann Dermato Venereol*; 132: 263–267.

Choi JY., Seo HM., Kim Ws.. (2017) Median canaliform nail dystrophy treated with z 1064-nm quasi -long pulsed Nd: YAG Laser. *J Cosmet Laser Ther*; 19: 225–226.

Deffer and Goette (1987) Distal phalangeal atrophy secondary to topical steroid therapy. *Arch Dermatol*; 123: 571–572.

Degreef I., de Smet L. (2007) Vanishing finger in psoriatic arthritis: a case report. *Clin Rheumatol*; 26: 1391–1392.

Dereure O., Camu W. (2017) Teriflunomide-induced psoriasiform changes of fingernails. *Int J Dermatol*; 56: 1479–1481.

Desanu CA., Argote JA., Lippman SM. et al. (2018) Longitudinal thumbnail fissures due to erlotinib therapy for lung cancer. *J Oncol Pharm Practice*; 24: 229–231.

Dharmagunawardena B., Charles-Holmès R. (1997) Median canaliform dystrophy following isotretinoin therapy. *Br J Dermatol*; 137: 658–659.

Keles MK., Yosma E., Aydogdu IO. et al. (2015) Multiple subungual pyogenic granulomas following levothyroxine treatment. *J Craniofac Surg*; 26: e476–e477.

Mancinelli L., Amerio P., di Loia M. et al. (2017) Nail loss after teriflunomide treatment: A new potential adverse event. *Multiple Sclerosis and Related Disorders*; 18: 170–172.

Martinez-de-Espronceda I., Barnabeu-Wittel J., Azcona M. et al. (2020) Recalcitrant Trametinib-induced paronychia treated successfully with topical timolol in a pediatric patient. *Dermatol Ther*; 33: e13164.

Mempanakit K., Geater A., Limtong P. et al. (2017) The use of topical minoxidil to accelerate nail growth: a pilot study. *Int J Dermatol*; 56: 788–791.

Panariello L., Donrarumma M., Cinelli E., Fabbrocini G. (2019) Case Series showing the efficacy of 5-aminolaevulinic acid Photodynamic therapy for epidermal growth factor receptor inhibitor-induced paronychia and pyogenic granuloma-like lesion. *Br J Dermatol*; 180: 676–677.

Piraccini BM., Alessandrini A., Dika E. et al. (2016) Topical propranolol 1% cream for pyogenic granulomas of the nail: open-label study in 10 patients. *JEADV*; 30: 901–902.

Sampson B., Lewis BKH. (2019) Paronychia associated with Ledipasvir/Sofosbuvir for Hepatitis C Treatment. *J Clin Aesthet Dermatol*; 12: 35–37.

Sari N. (2018) A possible rare side-effect due to tenofir: nail pitting. *Klimik Derg*; 31: 241–243.

Sibaud V., Casassa E., d'Andrea M. (2019) Are topical β-blockers really effective "in real life" for targeted therapy-induced paronychia? *Support care cancer*; 27: 2341–2343.

Tajalli M., Qureschi AA. (2019) Successful treatment of calcinosis cutis of fingertip in the setting of CREST syndrome with topical 20% sodium thiosulfate. *JAAD Case Reports*; 5: 988–989.

Tanenbaum MH. (1972) Topical steroid atrophy "A disappearing digit". *JAMA*; 220: 125.

Wolf R., Tur E., Brenner S. (1990) Corticosteroid-induced "Disappearing Digit". *J Am Acad Dermatol*; 23: 755–756.

Yen CF., Hsu CK., Lu CW. (2018) Topical betaxolol for treating relapsing paronychia with pyogenic granuloma-like lesions induced by epidermal growth factor receptor inhibitors. *JAAD*; 78: e 143–e 144.

Yorulmaz A., Yalcin B. (2020) Paronychia and periungual granulation as a novel side effect of Ibrutinib: a case report. *Skin Appendage Disorder*; 6: 32–36.

Zaraa I., Litaiem N., Zribi D. et al. (2013) Multiple eruptive periungual granuloma during risperidone therapy for schizophrenia. Marrakesh 2° ISND.

21

Classical nail surgery and removal of the proximal nail fold

Eckart Haneke
Robert Baran

A

Classical Nail Surgery

This short chapter is not intended to substitute a textbook of nail surgery but to give a short outline of the subject for daily dermatologic practice. In-depth knowledge of the anatomy and physiology of the nail is an absolute prerequisite for all types of nail surgeries (Figure 21.1).

Patient Selection

Nail surgeries are in almost all cases elective interventions. Patient selection has, therefore, to be carried out with care. Indications have to be cautiously weighed against potential risks. Peripheral circulatory impairment, microangiopathy, uncontroled diabetes mellitus, heavy smoking, and particularly infections of the nail unit are relative contraindications although surgery is sometimes the only means to cope with an infected nail. The patient is advised not to travel in the following days, particularly not into warm regions (Richert et al. 2011).

Patient Preparation

Patients should be aware of what will happen during and after surgery; thus, informed consent is a must. The digit to be operated should be scrubbed with a disinfective soap morning and evening starting 2 days prior to surgery. Smoking is to be interdicted, particularly on the day of operation. For toenail surgery, the patient is informed to bring an open shoe or sandal. Perioperative antibiotic prophylaxis may be discussed in case of delicate surgery and impossibility to completely sterilize the surgical field, particularly in case of bone surgery of the distal phalanx. The individual pain threshold is discussed in order to be able to adjust postoperative analgesics (Richert et al. 2011; Haneke 2017; Richert et al. 2019).

Anesthesia

Virtually all patients have a subconscious fear of nail surgery, not only of the needle prick for anesthesia. For nail surgery, a fast and long-acting anesthetic agent is highly recommended, e.g.,

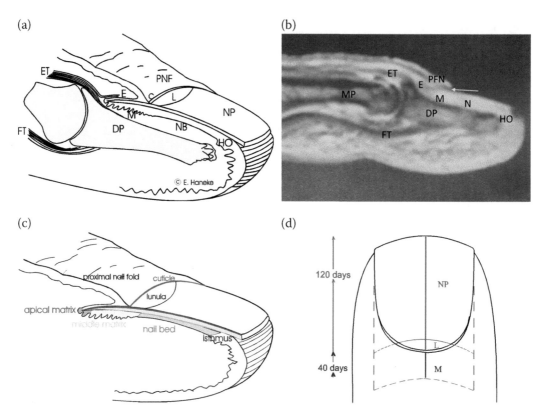

FIGURE 21.1 Surgical anatomy of the nail. (A) Schematic illustration of a sagittal section through the distal phalanx (C, Cuticle; DP, Distal phalanx; E, Eponychium; ET, Extensor tendon; FT, Flexor tendon; HO, Hyponychium; L, Lunula; M, Matrix; NB, Nail bed; NP, Nail plate; PNF, Proximal nail fold). (B) Magnetic resonance image of the distal phalanx of a middle finger. Most of the details from A are seen in B; however, the nail plate, cuticle, and lunula are not seen in the MRI; the arrow indicates the nail pocket (cul-de-sac). (C) Origin of the nail layers: Surface changes require a biopsy of the matrix, lesions in the nail plate from the mid-matrix whereas nail bed lesions remain under the nail. The nail isthmus is the most distal portion of the nail bed physiologically expressing a granular layer. (D) Growth characteristics of a fingernail: It takes about 40 days to grow from the apical matrix to the nail bed and another 3 months to the free margin.

ropivacaine. If this is not available 2% plain lidocaine is usually recommended although adrenaline 1:200,000 has been shown to prolong anesthesia without adverse effects in most cases (see Nail Surgery Complications). The higher the anesthetic concentration the faster is its onset and longer is its duration. The type of anesthesia varies according to the type of surgery to be performed and the surgeon's personal preferences; the lead author almost invariably uses a proximal digital block, but many nail surgeons use distal local anesthesia (Richert et al. 2011; Richert et al. 2019; Haneke 2017). For fingers 2–4, the transthecal anesthesia via the flexor tendon sheath is ideal (Figure 21.2) (Haneke 2017).

Hemostasis

If there is no real contraindication, it is strongly advised to use a tourniquet. Many different devices are available, from a simple rubber string to a wide metallic band. For fingernail surgery, a sterile glove is donned, a tiny hole cut at the tip of the finger, and the glove finger is then pulled over the tip and rolled down to the base of the finger; this maneuver yields a perfect exsanguination and tourniquet while giving a sterile surgical field for the entire hand. Another advantage is that the glove tourniquet will never be forgotten. Using a head magnifier loupe, vessel lumina less than 1 mm in diameter can be identified and ligated; bipolar electrocautery is sometimes used but there is a lot of heat destruction from this technique.

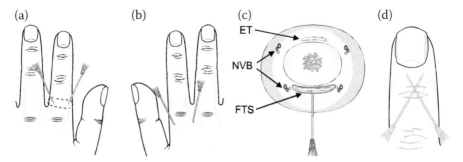

FIGURE 21.2   Anesthesia types for nail surgery. (A) Proximal finger block. (B) Metacarpal block. (C) Transthecal block for fingers 2–4 (ET, Extensor digitorum tendon; FTS, Flexor digitorum tendon; NVB, Neurovascular bundle). (D) So-called distal wing block.

When diffuse postoperative bleeding is expected, a hemostyptic solution, such as 30% aluminum chloride, may be used. A collagen fleece may be used as a pad for wound cavities that tend to bleed.

At the end of surgery, the wound is cleansed with 3% hydrogen peroxide, which dissolves the red blood cells and also has a strong antiseptic action (Haneke 2006).

Dressing

Dressings after nail surgery depend on the type of operation, localization, expected postoperative bleeding, patient's activities, the presumed period it will be left on, and particularly on personal preferences of the doctor or nurse applying them. I do all dressings myself, apply plenty of ointment and several layers of gauze to get a thick padded dressing that is able to take up blood and absorb shock. Whenever possible, the dressing is changed after 24 to 48 hours before the clotted blood is stone-hard; the wound is cleansed again with 3% hydrogen peroxide and a new dressing is performed. This may be a real bandage or just a tape depending on the type of wound (Haneke 2017; Richert et al. 2019).

Postoperative Management

Immediately after the dressing has been applied the operated extremity is elevated, which minimizes bleeding, inhibits swelling, prolongs the anesthetic action, and reduces overall pain during the entire healing phase. Analgesics are chosen according to the type of surgery, beginning with paracetamol or metamizole, adding codeine till tilidine. Certain operations involving the phalangeal bone may elicit extreme pain even after 24 hours, this is best treated with another anesthetic digital block.

Pain starting anew after 48 to 72 hours is usually a sign of infection. The dressing is removed to permit wound inspection and a swab is taken for bacterial culture and sensitivity testing. In case of obvious infection, skin sutures are removed and a staphylococcus-fast antibiotic is given; this is later adapted to the type of bacteria grown and their sensitivity (Haneke 2006, 2017).

Common Nail Surgeries

Except for cases where the intervention is aimed at reaching a diagnosis, no nail surgery must be performed without a working diagnosis. All interventions have to be carried out according to the principles of aesthetic surgery (Haneke 2017).

Nail Avulsion

Removing the nail plate is probably one of the most frequently performed surgeries worldwide – and the least indicated! It is almost never a treatment *per se* and must not be a substitute of a diagnosis. Different techniques are described in the surgical literature, but many are very crude and often result in permanent nail dystrophy. The technique using a sturdy hemostat clamp, running it under the proximal nail fold and then under the nail, firmly grasping the plate and tearing it from the nail bed by rotating the hemostat clamp is extremely traumatizing and, therefore, obsolete. There are two recommended techniques using a blunt nail elevator: the distal and the proximal approach (Figure 21.3).

In the *distal nail avulsion*, the slightly bent elevator with its tip pointing down to the nail plate is inserted under the proximal fold and pushed proximally to the blind end of the cul-de-sac; this is repeated from one side to the other. The elevator is then pushed under the nail through the hyponychium to the end of the matrix with its tip pointing upward to the nail again from one side to the other, freeing the nail completely from its attachments. In the *proximal avulsion* approach, the nail is freed from the overlying nail fold, and the tip of the elevator is then slipped under the proximal end of the nail plate along the matrix and nail bed to the hyponychium detaching the nail entirely from one side to the other. This technique is the least traumatizing as it does not tear nail bed epithelium from its dermis. However, as mentioned above, nail avulsion alone is not a treatment, except for retronychia, but the beginning of a therapy of either the matrix, nail bed or both (Haneke 2011).

Diagnostic Biopsies (Figure 21.4a–d)

Histopathology is the diagnostic gold standard of nail disorders. It requires a good biopsy from the correct site, a dermatopathology lab experienced in handling nail specimens, and a pathologist familiar with skin and nail disorders. These triple demands are unfortunately not often met as nail biopsies are not performed often enough (Haneke 2015).

1. *Nail plate biopsies* are simple nail clippings and when performed correctly, allow the diagnosis of onychomycoses and psoriasis, often of nail eczema and alopecia areata to be made or ruled out. It is of utmost importance that the clipping contains as much of subungual keratosis as possible. The specimen does not need fixation and can be sent dry to the lab. Parallel direct microscopy after KOH clearing and mycologic culture is recommended.

2. *Biopsy of the proximal nail fold* may be helpful in the diagnosis of collagen diseases if this site would be the only unequivocal site of clinical alterations. However, care has to be taken as wound healing may be considerably impaired.

3. *Tzanck test* from blisters of the nail folds may be useful for the diagnosis of digital herpes simplex and pemphigus vulgaris.

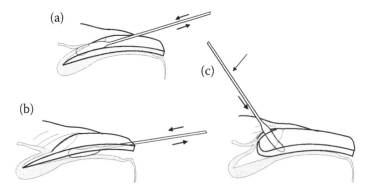

FIGURE 21.3   Distal and proximal approach of nail avulsion. (A) First step: separation of the proximal nail fold from the underlying nail plate. (B) Separation of the nail plate from the underlying nail bed via the hyponychium in the distal approach. (C) Detachment of the nail from the matrix and nail bed via the proximal matrix in the proximal approach.

4. *Nail bed biopsies* may be performed as a 3 mm to maximally 4 mm punch, with the nail plate or after nail avulsion. *Fusiform nail bed biopsies* are performed after avulsion and always in the longitudinal axis of the nail bed. They may be 4–5 mm long and up to 2 mm wide and can thus be directly sutured with fast-absorbing stitches (Figure 21.4).

5. *Matrix biopsies* are indicated for unclear changes of the nail surface and nail dystrophies. Depending on the presumed localization of the pathologic process, a 3 mm punch may be directly taken from the lunula without interfering with its border to the nail bed. If the lesion is localized more proximally in the matrix, the proximal nail fold is incised on both sides and detached from the underlying nail plate revealing the site of biopsy. The nail plate is partially removed in case of a narrow fusiform biopsy, which has to be oriented transversely in order to prevent a post-biopsy split nail.

6. Laterally localized lesions may be biopsied or excised using a *lateral longitudinal nail biopsy*. This starts at the distal interphalangeal joint crease 2 mm median from the lateral nail plate margin down to the bone through the matrix and nail bed to the hyponychium. The second longitudinal incision starts again from the joint and extends straight through the lateral sulcus to the hyponychium. The proximal incision may be slightly slanted outwards to avoid leaving pieces of the lateral matrix horn behind. The entire narrow tissue block is dissected from the bone using pointed curved iris scissors. Simple stitches are used for the wound in the proximal nail fold and backstitches in the level of the proximal nail bed to elevate the lateral nail fold (Richert et al. 2011; Haneke 2017). This biopsy gives information about all parts of the nail unit that may have occurred in the last 6 months or more. The lateral longitudinal biopsy may also be adapted for the removal of laterally localized nail tumors.

7. The *tangential matrix and nail bed biopsy* was developed for the diagnosis of melanocytic foci giving rise to longitudinal melanonychia and can also be used for superficial lesions of the nail bed such as onychopapilloma. Depending on the exact localization in the matrix or nail bed and type of lesion, a variable approach is recommended. For matrix lesions, such as a melanocytic nevus or early melanoma, the proximal nail fold is incised on both sides, detached from the underlying nail plate and reclined. The nail is cut transversely from one side to about 3 mm beyond and 5 mm distal of the lesion and carefully separated from the matrix; this piece is lifted up like a trapdoor exposing the lesion. Using a #15 scalpel, a shallow incision with an adequate safety margin is made around it and a horizontal – tangential excision is made with saw-like movements of the scalpel yielding a specimen with a thickness of 0.8–1 mm. The matrix tissue is very soft and a very sharp ophthalmic blade should be used. If the lesion is located in the nail bed, an analogous technique is used. For onychopapillomas, the overlying nail may be avulsed facilitating the tangential excision, or the nail plate may be longitudinally incised on both sides and the lesion horizontally removed *en bloc*; this, however, requires experience with the technique.

Ingrown Toenails

There are many different types of ingrowing nails that are more or less characteristic for certain age periods.

1. Distal and distal-lateral *ingrown nails in neonates* are treated conservatively. The mother takes the baby, puts the foot, after applying plenty of vaseline, into warm water and gently massages the distal and lateral nail folds away from the nail. Within a few days, the nail has enough space to grow out without further complication. A similar approach is also effective in many cases of the *hypertrophic lateral lip*, in which a grossly hypertrophic medial nail fold lies on the nail plate (Arai et al. 2010).

2. *Congenital malalignment of the big toenail* is not so uncommon as often believed. It is characterized by a lateral deviation of the nail's long axis relative to that of the distal phalanx. The nail is obliquely inserted, discolored, thickened, oyster shell-like, triangular, medially bent, and severely onycholytic (Baran and Haneke 1998). There is a distal bulge and a markedly shortened nail bed. The degree of onycholysis and nail bed shortening define the prognosis. In fact, without onycholysis the nail may look normal even despite a marked lateral deviation. The condition is virtually always associated with a hallux valgus interphalangeal plus common type of hallux valgus. A certain percentage of congenital malalignment cases may resolve spontaneously, but this is not observed when the onycholysis is pronounced. Treatment should start as early as possible. The toe is taped to correct the hallux valgus

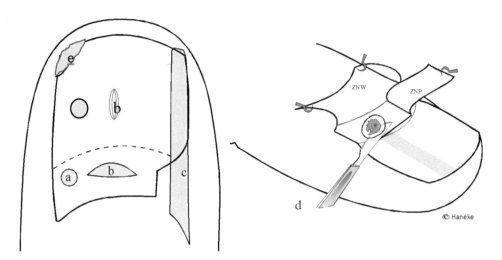

FIGURE 21.4   Nail biopsy techniques. (A) Punch biopsy: matrix maximal diameter 3 mm, nail bed maximal diameter 4 mm; (B) Fusiform biopsy: transverse orientation in matrix, longitudinal orientation in nail bed; (C) Lateral longitudinal nail biopsy: starts proximal of the apical matrix, runs through the nail to its free margin and hyponychium, then the second incision runs parallel to first one right next to the lateral nail plate margin; (D) Tangential nail matrix (and nail bed) biopsy after refection of the proximal nail fold and the proximal half of the nail plate; (E) Nail plate biopsy.

interphalangeal, the nail plate is pulled medially and fixed with tape, and the distal bulge is pulled down with tape. This has to be done every day for as long as possible, particularly during daytime when the baby crawls and walks. This often improves the nail appearance considerably. When this therapy is ineffective a surgical redirection of the entire nail unit is necessary. A fish-mouth incision is performed around the distal phalanx approximately 5–6 mm below the level of the nail bed, a second incision is made to yield a horizontal wedge of soft tissue to be removed, which permits flattening of the distal bulge. The entire nail unit, including the lateral matrix horns, are dissected from the bone, rotated into the axis of the phalanx and sutured in orthograde position (Baran and Haneke 1998). Sometimes, the distal phalangeal bone is also heaped up dorsally and has to be flattened. Healing has been uneventful in all cases and postoperative pain appears to be surprisingly low. The success rate is about 50%.

3. *Adolescent type of ingrown nail* is the most common Figure 21.5a–b.) It affects school children, adolescents, and young adults. The distal lateral margin of the nail pierces into the lateral nail sulcus and elicits an acute to chronic inflammation with granulation tissue. There may be perilesional erythema and swelling. Antibiotics are often given although it is the ingrown nail that causes this condition and bacterial colonization is only secondary.

   3a. There are several conservative means to treat ingrown nails: Pulling the soft tissue away from the offending nail margin with tape (taping), inserting a wisp of cotton between the nail and the soft tissue (packing), freeing the soft tissue from the nail with dental floss, flattening the overcurved nail with braces from plastic or steel or with shape memory alloy clips, and many more. These techniques require strict coherence to the treatment details and meticulous nail care after resolution of the acute symptoms. A semiconservative treatment is the insertion of a gutter over the ingrown lateral nail margin and fixing with tape, suture, or acrylic glue.

   If the patient is not able or willing to perform a long-term conservative therapy, surgery is indicated (Arai et al. 2010).

   There are two fundamentally different approaches: Those believing that a wide nail is at fault will narrow the nail, those convinced the hypertrophic nail folds are causative will reduce the folds (Haneke 2012).

   3b. Selective lateral matrix horn removal, either by scalpel, laser vaporization, radio surgery, or chemocautery, is the surgery of choice. The ingrown side of the nail is freed from the proximal nail fold and nail bed, cut longitudinally and avulsed. The matrix horn is then cauterized with liquefied phenol three times for 1 minute under complete anemia achieved with a tourniquet. Excessive granulation tissue may be phenolized or curetted. Postoperative pain and morbidity are very low. This operation is quick, easy and time-honoring. Long-term success rates are >98%, recurrences are very rare. However, the matrix horn may also be destroyed with 10% sodium hydroxide, 85–100% trichloroacetic acid, CO_2 laser or radiosurgery; the results are comparable and do not depend on the means by which the matrix horn is removed, but by the experience of the surgeon (Haneke 2012).

3c. When the nail folds are excessively hypertrophic, they may be radically reduced by excision, again with various techniques. Vandenbos procedure starts the excision in the lateral aspect of the proximal nail fold and excises till the border of the lateral third to the mid-third of the hyponychium, just leaving a bridge of one-third of the hyponychium. Perez Rosa's super-U excises both lateral folds plus the entire hyponychium. There are many variants in radicality and design, but they should all have in common not to touch the matrix. Postoperative morbidity is significant and healing is by secondary intention that takes weeks to months, but the long-term results are good (Haneke 2017, 2012).

3d. Wedge excisions, including part of the matrix, nail bed, and nail fold are still the most frequently performed operations for ingrown nails worldwide. However, if their design is wrong, the recurrence rates are between 25% and 70%, postoperative pain and morbidity are high. Wedge excisions are, therefore, obsolete (Haneke, 2012).

Removal of the Proximal Nail Fold

Experience of biopsy material from the proximal nail fold (PNF) (Baran and Bureau 1991) for example for collagen diseases (Figure 21.6a–b) has suggested a surgical approach for the treatment of recalcitrant chronic paronychia.

An excision of a crescent-shaped full-thickness skin bevelled upside – 4–5 mm at its greatest width from one lateral nail fold to the other and including most of the entire swollen portion of the PNF – is performed (Figure 21.7a–b). Complete healing by secondary intention takes about one month.

In patients who experience repeated acute painful flares associated with chronic paronychia, removal of the base of the nail plate is useful, total nail avulsion being rarely necessary.

The latest surgical technique imagined by a Brazilian team removes only the core of the fibrotic tissue of the proximal and lateral nail folds and obtains optimal cosmetic results (Ferreira Vieira d'Almeida et al. 2016).

Some tumors involving the distal PNF may be treated with this crescent technique.

Micronychia may benefit from a crescent-shaped full-thickness nail fold removal in order to increase the length of the nail.

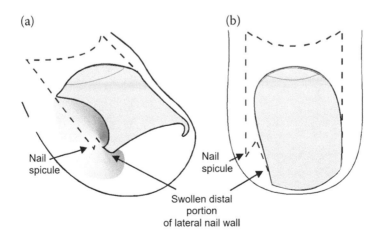

(a)   (b)

Nail spicule

Nail spicule

Swollen distal portion of lateral nail wall

FIGURE 21.5   Adolescent type of ingrown toenail: (A) Oblique view; (B) Dorsal view.

(a)   (b)

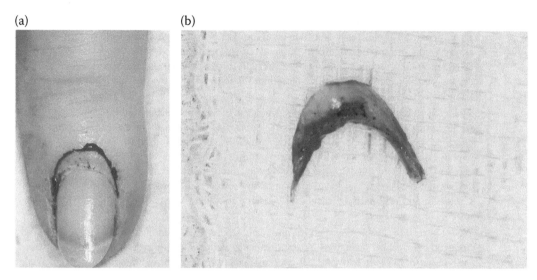

FIGURE 21.6   (a) Biopsy of the distal proximal nail fold; (b) Material removed.

Recreation of the PNF

When only partially torn, recreation of the PNF can be managed by excising its remaining portion to get a uniform crescent shaped.

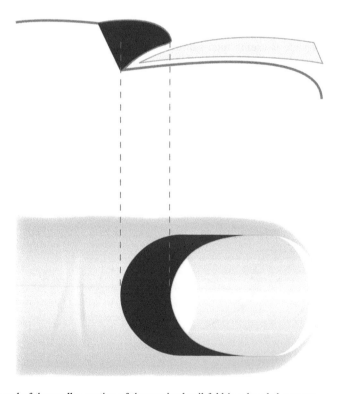

FIGURE 21.7   Removal of the swollen portion of the proximal nail fold in a beveled manner.

- Nail surgery requires exact knowledge of the nail's anatomy and physiology as well as surgical skills and atraumatic surgery.
- Patients have to be prepared before surgery and be given information as to what to expect after surgery: pain, inability to work and perform sports, etc.
- Detailed information for postoperative management has to be given.
- Sufficient and long-lasting anesthesia is a must.
- An infected nail is usually not operated.
- Nail avulsion is unnecessary in most cases and often does more harm than good.
- There are many options to treat ingrown toenails with phenolization being the easiest and most efficacious.

BIBLIOGRAPHY

Arai H., Arai T., Haneke E. (2010) Simple and effective conservative treatment for ingrowing nails (Acrylic affixed gutter splint, sculptured nail and anchor taping methods). *Rinsho Derma (Tokyo)*; 52(11): 1604–1613.

Baran R., Bureau H. (1991) Surgical treatment of recalcitrant chronic paronychia. *J. Dermatol Surg Oncol*; 7: 106–107.

Baran R., Haneke E. (1998) Etiology and treatment of nail malalignment. *Dermatol Surg*; 24: 719–721.

Ferreira Vieira d'Almeida L., Papaiordanou F, Araujo Machado E. et al. (2016) Chronic paronychia treatment: square flap technique. *JAAD*; 75:398–03.

Haneke E. (2006) Nail surgery: indications and outcome. *Expert Rev Dermatol*; 1: 93–104.

Haneke E. (2011) Advanced nail surgery. *J Cutan Aesthet Surg*; 4: 167–175.

Haneke E. (2012) Controversies in the treatment of ingrown nails. *Dermatol Res Pract*; 1–12 Article ID 783924, doi:10.1155/2012/783924.

Haneke E. (2015) Anatomy of the nail unit and the nail biopsy. *Semin Cutan Med Surg*; 34: 95–100.

Haneke E. (2017) Nail surgery. In André P, Haneke E, Marini L, Rowland Payne C *Cosmetic Dermatology and Surgery*. Taylor & Francis CRC Press, London, 287–302.

Richert B., Di Chiacchio N., Haneke E. (2011) *Nail Surgery*. Informa healthcare, New York – London.

Richert B., Haneke E., Zook E. G., Baran R (2019) Nail surgery. In Baran & Dawber's *Diseases of the Nails and their Management*. 5th ed. Wiley Blackwell, London, 825–895.

22

Surgery of some common nail tumors

Eckart Haneke

Fibrokeratoma

Ungual fibrokeratomas are sausage-shaped tumors arising from the depth of the nail pocket and lying on the nail (Figure 21.1), from the matrix and growing for a certain period in the nail plate, or from the nail bed and growing under the nail. Surgery is the treatment of choice. A pointed scalpel is held parallel to the tumor and carried around the base of the fibroma down to the bone, from which it is dissected with a pair of pointed sharp iris scissors. The small wound rapidly heals by secondary intention without leaving a visible scar or nail dystrophy (Richert et al. 2011, 2006; Haneke 2017, 2006).

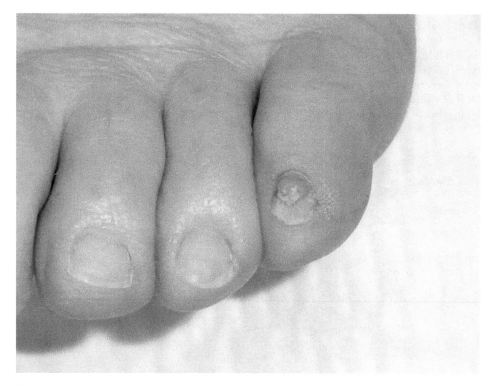

FIGURE 22.1   Fibrokeratoma.

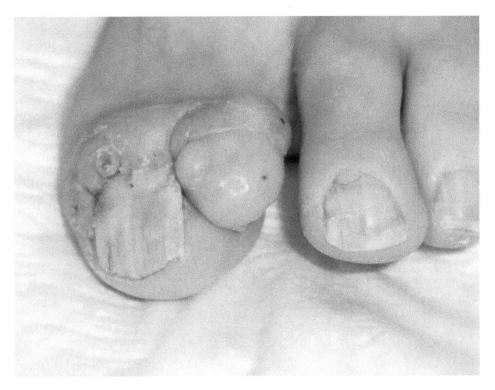

FIGURE 22.2   Koenen's tumors.

Koenen's tumors of tuberous sclerosis (Figure 21.2) are histologically alike fibrokeratomas. In principle, their treatment is the same as that of acquired fibrokeratomas; however, they are often multiple and can no longer be removed singly. When they are disturbing, the nail is avulsed and the lesions are cut at their base, but they may recur. An alternative is to cut the multiple fibrokeratomas at the level of the nail and use phenol or CO_2 laser on the remaining base of the Koenen tumors. Sirolimus as used for facial angiofibromas may be a therapeutic option in these cases (Haneke 2017).

Myxoid Pseudocyst

There are many synonyms for this frequent degenerative lesion of the proximal nail fold of fingers and rarely toes, reflecting the different opinions as to its etiopathogenesis. In the beginning, a circumscribed mucinosis is seen that develops to a lake of mucin, which, in turn, compresses the surrounding fibroblasts, thus forming a pseudo-capsule, however, without an epithelial lining. With time, a connection with the distal interphalangeal joint may develop. Three clinical types are differentiated: Type A (Figure 21.3) is seen as a dome-shaped, round, rubbery, elastic nodule pressing on the matrix and causing a regular longitudinal depression (Figure 21.4) in the nail; type B is also in the nail fold but tends to rupture into the cul-de-sac with consecutive irregular longitudinally arranged depressions; type C (Figure 21.5) is under the matrix and seen as a violaceous lunula with hemi overcurvature of the nail and positive transillumination. There are many different treatment approaches: Repeated needling and

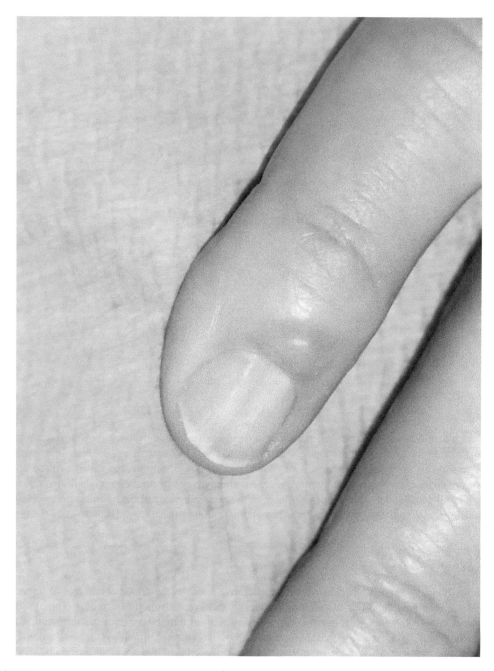

FIGURE 22.3   Myxoid pseudocyst, Type A.

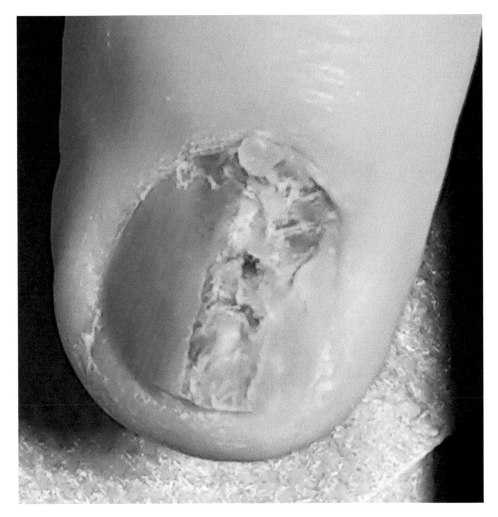

FIGURE 22.4   Myxoid pseudocyst, Type B.

expression of the content with consecutive long-term pressure is sometimes sufficient. Alternatively, the content may be expressed and either a steroid crystal suspension or a sclerosing agent such as 1% aethoxysclerol injected with a several week-long compression. Laser vaporization, infrared coagulation or cryotherapy are further possibilities. If these simple methods are unsuccessful, surgical removal is advocated. Simple excision and suture are almost invariably followed by a recurrence. Depending on the viability of the overlying skin, this is either raised as a U-shaped flap or excised and the lesion is meticulously dissected. Preoperative intraarticular methylene blue injection makes a potential stalk to the joint visible and also stains the mucinous content blue. If a dark-blue spot is seen indicating a connection to the joint, this is ligated like a bleeding artery. The raised flap is laid back or a transposition flap is raised and used to cover the primary defect; the secondary defect rapidly heals by secondary

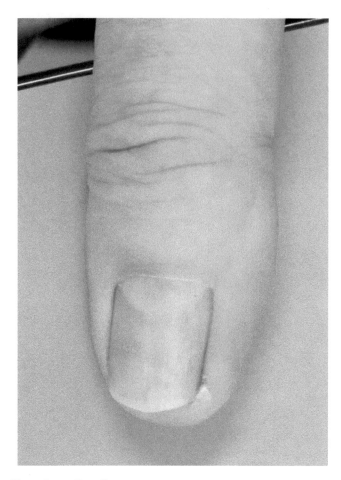

FIGURE 22.5   Myxoid pseudocyst, Type C.

intention. Submatrical pseudocysts are either punctured and injected or dissected after partial nail plate avulsion. These surgical techniques have a success rate of > 80% and almost no postoperative stiffening of the distal interphalangeal joint, which is the major risk of exclusive removal of Heberden nodes (Haneke 2017, 2011).

Subungual Exostosis

Subungual exostosis (Figure 21.6) is a relatively common lesion mostly seen under the big toenail in children and young adults. The nail is lifted up on one corner by a tumor that has a very smooth shiny surface, is stone-hard on palpation, and exhibits a very characteristic collarette-like margin, which represents the border between the pulp skin and nail bed. Ulceration may occur with time. Pain is exceptional. The diagnosis is confirmed by radiography, which also allows the entire extent of the

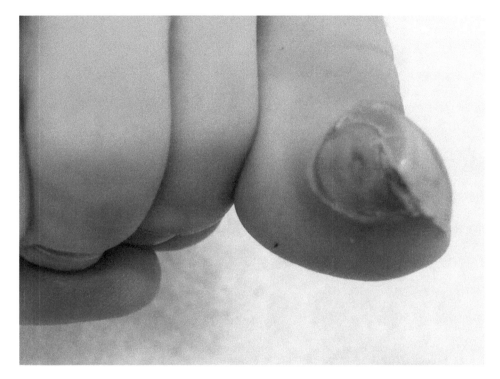

FIGURE 22.6   Subungual exostosis.

exostosis to be seen; this is important as remnants of the base when left behind may cause recurrences. Subungual exostoses were believed to be reactive to chronic repeated trauma as they were frequently observed in ballet dancers, kick boxers, and other persons performing martial arts sports; however, as investigations demonstrated a tumor-specific chromosomal translocation t(X genes;6)(q14-14;q22) with a rearrangement of COL12A1 and COL4A5 a true neoplasm was suggested (Haneke 2017; Richert et al. 2019; Haneke 2011).

Glomus Tumor

This relatively rare benign neoplasm is the best-known nail tumor because of its very characteristic symptomatology of extreme tenderness to slight pressure, mild shock, and cold. It is usually seen as a violaceous round to oval spot in the distal matrix, from which a reddish band extends along the nail bed to the hyponychium (Figure 21.7). Using a blunt probe usually allows the exact localization of the lesion even if it is smaller than the resolution of magnetic resonance imaging, which is otherwise the preferred diagnostic measure (Figure 21.8). Laterally localized glomus tumors can be extirpated via an L-shaped incision of the side of the phalanx and pulp approximately 5 mm below the level of the nail bed, which is then dissected until the glomus tumor is reached that stands out by its greyish-glassy appearance in contrast to the white of the nail bed and matrix dermis. If the glomus tumor is located more medially, the overlying nail is lifted, and a slightly curved superficial incision is made extending 2 mm beyond the

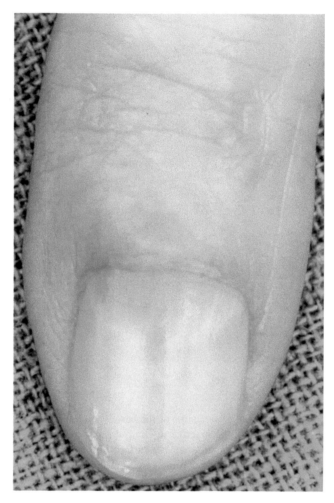

FIGURE 22.7 A glomus tumor in the lunular area with longitudinal erythronychia.

visible bluish spot in the matrix or a longitudinal incision in the nail bed. The epithelium with a thin layer of dermis is cautiously dissected from the underlying greyish tumor that is clearly discernable. The incision line is closed with fast absorbable 6-0 stitches and the nail plate is laid back. As no matrix or nail bed epithelium is excised a normal nail will regrow (Haneke 2011; Duarte et al. 2016).

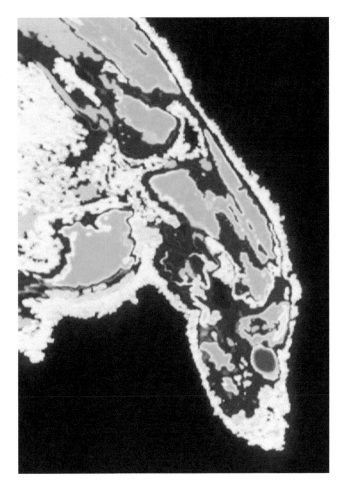

FIGURE 22.8   Color-coded MRI of a subungual glomus tumor.

Erythronychia

Erythronychia describes a red nail, in most cases as a longitudinal red line under or in the nail, more rarely red spots or a red lunula. The latter are mainly inflammatory or vascular in origin, whereas the former are due to a variety of other causes, such as lichen planus (Figure 21.9). Multiple red lines may be isolated or seen in dyskeratosis follicularis of Darier or in keratosis cristarum. Erythronychia is sometimes associated with onychopapilloma (Figure 21.10). The latter and subungual Bowen's disease (see below) are single lesions and of epithelial origin, whereas the red streak distal to a glomus tumor is thought to be vascular. Onychopapilloma is best excised in a longitudinal tangential way (see above Chapter Biopsy). This may be done after cautious nail plate avulsion or include the overlying nail. It is important to note that the onychopapilloma stretches from the mid-matrix to the hyponychium and that the tangential excision must not be too superficial as this is associated with a higher recurrence rate (Haneke 2017, 2011). Bowen's disease requires a diagnostic biopsy for diagnosis and subsequent

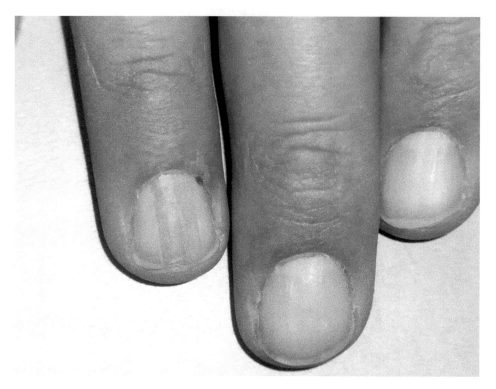

FIGURE 22.9   Lichen planus presenting as longitudinal erythronychia in a single digit.

adequate therapy, best by microscopically controlled surgery (Perruchoud et al. 2016). The biopsy techniques for multiple red lines and erythematous spots depend on their localization and size (see above).

Longitudinal Melanonychia

A brown to black streak in the nail may be caused by a variety of pigments. If it is due to melanin, the brown color reaches into the free margin of the nail plate as its cause is either melanocytic hyperactivity or melanocyte hyperplasia in the matrix (Figure 21.11). The color itself does not allow the identity of the etiologic lesion to be determined. Treatment of single longitudinal melanonychia is best by tangential excision of the matrix lesion with an adequate safety margin (see above) (Haneke and Baran 2001; Haneke 2012), while polydactylous melanonychia is centered on a search for underlying local, regional or systemic causes.

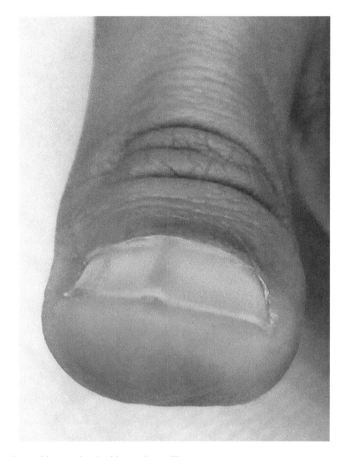

FIGURE 22.10   Erythronychia associated with onychopapilloma.

Ungual Bowen's Disease

This is said to be the most frequent malignancy of the nail (Figure 21.12). Most cases occur in middle-aged to elderly men on thumb, index and middle fingers, rarely on toes suggesting a genito-digital transmission. Its growth is slow and insidious, usually beginning in the lateral sulcus and extending under the nail. Matrix involvement causes leukonychia or nail dystrophy, rarely erythronychia. Most ungual Bowen's cases are associated with high-risk HPV (Perruchoud et al. 2016) The involved skin is reddish to hyperkeratotic to verrucous, but the delimitation is often not clear. The true extent can be estimated by photodynamic diagnosis. The treatment of choice is complete excision with three-dimensional margin control (Richert et al. 2011). Laterally localized Bowen's disease may simulate a fibrokeratoma and is removed by segmental excision (Haneke 2017). When more than half of the nail is involved a total nail ablation is preferable (Haneke 2011).

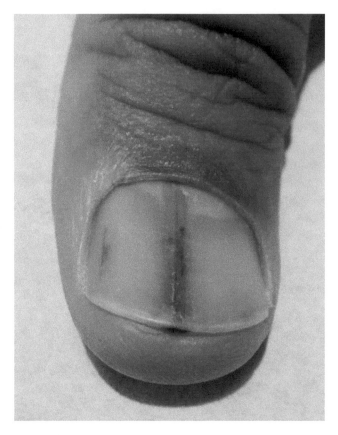

FIGURE 22.11 Longitudinal melanonychia.

Ungual Squamous Cell Carcinoma (SCC)

By far most of ungual SCCs develop from Bowen's disease and have a long history (Figure 21.13). Invasive SCC is commonly marked by malodorous oozing onycholysis. Treatment is complete extirpation with three-dimensional margin control (Richert et al. 2011; Haneke 2017, 2011) Preoperative radiography has not shown better results.

Ungual Melanoma

Melanoma of the nail unit makes up for about 2% of all melanomas in light-skinned Caucasians (Figure 21.14), but up to 20%–30% in Blacks and Asians; however, in absolute numbers, nail

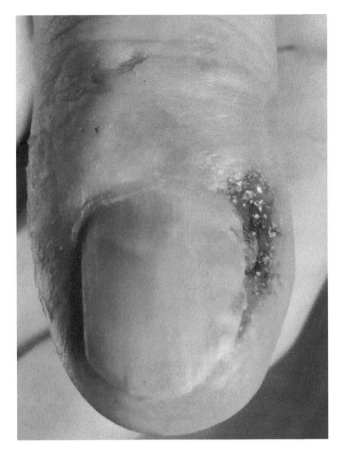

FIGURE 22.12 Bowen's carcinoma.

melanomas occur at the same rate in the various races. Two-thirds of ungual melanomas are pigmented, one quarter to one third are amelanotic (Haneke 2012; Duarte et al. 2016). Most amelanotic melanomas arise from the nail bed, most matrix melanoma are pigmented. Primary periungual melanomas are very rare, but periungual pigmentation in the course of melanoma development represents *in situ* spread of subungual melanoma. Treatment of primary nail melanoma is complete surgical removal. *In situ* and early invasive melanomas are adequately treated by total extirpation of the entire nail unit with a 5–6 mm margin around the anatomical borders of the nail apparatus (Haneke 2012) As so-called field cells have been found up to 9 mm from the visible margin of *in situ* acral lentiginous melanomas the safety margin around Hutchinson's sign is 10 mm (Duarte et al. 2016; Duarte et al. 2010). The defect may be left for secondary intention healing or grafted with split or full-thickness skin; the best results are achieved with guided wound healing and grafting after granulation tissue has reached the level of the previous nail bed (Duarte et al. 2010) Frankly invasive ungual melanomas are still treated with amputation; however, there is no unanimity as to the level of amputation, sentinel lymph node extirpation, and adjuvant therapies (Haneke 2012).

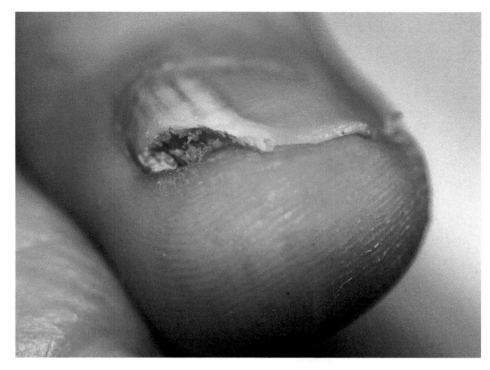

FIGURE 22.13   Squamous cell carcinoma. (By courtesy of L. Thomas, France.)

- Ungual fibrokeratomas are excised down to the bone.
- Myxoid pseudocysts may be injected or carefully extirpated.
- Glomus tumors are removed via a lateral or transungual approach.
- Subungual exostoses should be extirpated without leaving remnants of their base.
- Erythronychia may represent onychopapilloma or be a sign of Bowen's disease.
- Longitudinal melanonychia is best diagnosed using a tangential excisional biopsy.
- Most nail melanomas do not require an amputation.

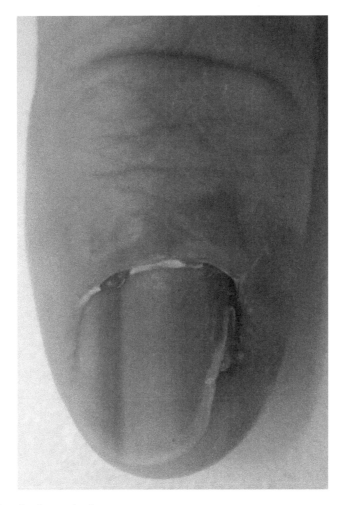

FIGURE 22.14   Ungual melanoma in situ.

REFERENCES

Duarte A. F., Correia O., Barros A. M., Azevedo R., Haneke E. (2010) Nail matrix melanoma in situ: conservative surgical management. *Dermatology* 220: 173–175.

Duarte A. F., Correia O., Barreiros H., Haneke E. (2016) Giant subungual glomus tumor: clinical, dermoscopy, imagiologic and surgery details. *Dermatol Online J*; 22(10). pii: 13030/qt66f7b8wt.

Haneke E. (2006) Nail surgery: indications and outcome. *Expert Rev Dermatol*; 1: 93–104.

Haneke, E. (2011) Advanced nail surgery. *J Cutan Aesthet Surg*; 4: 167–175.

Haneke E. (2012) Ungual melanoma – controversies in diagnosis and treatment. *Dermatol Ther*; 25: 510–524

Haneke E. (2017) Nail surgery. In André P, Haneke E, Marini L, Rowland Payne C (eds) *Cosmetic Dermatology and Surgery*. Taylor & Francis CRC Press, London 287–302.

Haneke E., Baran R. (2001) Longitudinal melanonychia. *Dermatol Surg*; 27: 580–584.

Perruchoud D. L., Varonier C., Haneke E., Hunger R. E., Beltraminelli H., Borradori L., Ehnis Pérez A. (2016) Bowen disease of the nail unit: a retrospective study of 12 cases and their association with human papillomaviruses. *J Eur Acad Dermatol Venereol*; 30: 1503–1506.

Richert B., Di Chiacchio N., Haneke E. (eds) (2011) *Nail Surgery*. Informa Healthcare, New York, London.

Richert B., Haneke E., Zook E. G., Baran R. (2019) Nail surgery. In *Baran & Dawber's Diseases of the Nails and their Management* (eds) 5th ed. Wiley Blackwell, London, 825–895.

23

Nail surgery complications

Robert Baran
Eckart Haneke

All types of nail surgery, whether diagnostic or therapeutic, should take into account both the functional aspect and the cosmetic appearance. Perfect knowledge of the nail anatomy and its pathology is crucial. Nail surgery is usually performed using local anesthesia and, in most cases, a tourniquet. Epinephrine is not used with a tourniquet, in young children, heavy smokers, and elderly persons (arterial impairment). The volume and concentration are adjusted according to age, size, and general condition. Ropivacaine is the ideal drug as its onset is as fast as that of lidocaine and its duration as long as that of bupivacaine.

Surgery of the nail is not recommended in high-risk patients, but the importance of systemic disease in nail abnormalities and of risk factors for nail surgery is often overemphasized. Infection is a contraindication except surgery is its treatment.

A history of concomitant administration of drugs may be relevant. Monoamine oxidase inhibitors or phenothiazines may affect anesthesia, steroids, and cytostatic agents delay healing, retinoids, and others have toxic effects on the nail. Prolonged bleeding due to aspirin or anticoagulants is rarely a problem as nail surgery is performed under a tourniquet and major arterial bleeding is virtually not possible.

Allergy to lidocaine, mepivacaine and other amide type local anesthetics is very rare; if this is suspected, articaine may be used. They contain parabens as preservative.

Anxiety before Nail Surgery

Anxiety is due to fear of needle prick and heightens the perception of pain; hydroxyzine taken at bedtime the day before surgery and a short-life benzodiazepine sublingually 1 hour prior to surgery are very effective. In those patients who are extremely anxious, squeezing a stress ball with the free hand does not interfere with the surgical procedure. The physician may use a hand-held vibrating massager placed directly on the digit proximal to the site of local anesthetic injection, causing further neurodistraction by the gate theory (Clark and Jellinek 2016). EMLA cream alleviates the pain of the needle prick and buffered lidocaine the burn sensation produced by infusion of the anesthetic. Ropivacaine is painless, acts immediately, and has a long duration of action (>6 hours), as well as the benefit of some intrinsic vasoconstriction. The addition of epinephrine, if there are no contra-indications, prolongs the anesthetic effect of lidocaine, thus alleviating postoperative pain. The addition of 0.4 mg dexamethasone in the original anesthesia site, if there is no infection, may reduce swelling.

Acute Complications Following Local Anesthesia

Pain and Swelling

Prevention

- Higher concentrations of the anesthetic and long-acting anesthetics (ropivacaine, if not available bupivacaine) offer postoperative analgesia for up to 16 hours.

- Painkillers are prescribed according to the expected postoperative pain. Some procedures cause very little pain (chemical cautery, debulking), whereas some others are very painful (wedge excision, DuBois Z-plasty).
- The operated digit is very sensitive to touch post-surgery and should be judiciously protected against trauma with a bulky dressing.
- To prevent swelling that will promote pain and throbbing, elevate the limb for 48 hours (arm sling or footstool) and avoid too tight a dressing.

If all recommendations mentioned above are carefully followed, postoperative pain is usually well tolerated by patients.

- If pain is still intolerable after 24 hours, a second digital block with ropivacaine is strongly recommended.
- If there is still major pain after 48 hours, perform an x-ray and rule out any infection.

Intra-operative pain is due to improper anesthesia or insufficient time allowed for the anesthesia to work. Pain was reported at some point during Mohs micrographic surgery, especially by patients who spent a long time in the office; they have to be re-injected. Additional preventive measures may be considered in patients at higher risk (Connolly et al. 2016).

Very important: etiologic factors should be looked for and pain may be treated with (1) analgesics for relatively **low perceived levels of pain** (paracetamol, non-steroidal anti-inflammatory drug [NSAID]); (2) weak opioids when pain is **moderately perceived** (codeine, tramadol associated with the previous pain killers); (3) strong opioids in presence of **intense pain.**

Dysesthesia

Occurrence of postoperative long-term dysesthesia after nail surgery is well known. Complete or partial resolution may be observed after several months.

A sensory disturbance was observed in about half of the patients without any relationship to the extent of the surgery undertaken. The most reported sensations were numbness or loss of sensation and tingling. When mapping the location of altered sensation, the digit tip was the most commonly affected with the proximal nail fold and margin beneath the free edge of the nail. Complete or partial resolution was noted in one-third of cases after 6 to 12 months.

TABLE 23.1

Recommended Safe Doses of Local Anesthetics

Anesthetic agent	Solution without adrenaline	Solution with adrenaline
Lidocaine	500 mg	700 mg
	7 mg/kg	10 mg/kg
Mepivacaine	400 mg	400 mg
	5–6 mg/kg	5–6 mg/kg
Ropivacaine	225 mg	
	3 mg/kg	
Bupivacaine	150 mg	180 mg
	2 mg/kg	2.5 mg/kg
Levo-bupivacaine	200 mg	
	3 mg/kg	

Bleeding

Above all, use a **tourniquet** because "operating on a hand without a tourniquet is like trying to fix a watch in a bottle of black ink" (Cox and Yao 2012). Intra-operative bleeding requires to check the tourniquet.

Postoperative bleeding within the wound may very rarely lead to hematoma.

At the end of surgery, use 35% aluminum chloride and oxidized cellulose or a gelatin sponge-saturated with the solution, which has been shown to assist in hemostasis during nail procedures (Howe and Cherpelis 2013). However, as the vessels involved are small, the bleeding can usually be controlled by direct pressure. For severe bleeding, injection of some anesthetic as a wing block of bupivacaine will act as a volumetric tourniquet. Electrosurgery is not recommended in nail surgery as it destroys a lot of tissue. Nevertheless, it can cause complications in patients with implantable devices; bipolar electrocautery avoids major risks to sensitive implants.

Infection

Knowledge of previous anti-tetanus immunization is important because administration of tetanus toxoid may be advisable in association with surgery involving the toenail or traumatic lesions that have come into contact with soil.

Osteitis should be feared in case of postoperative superinfection.

Prevention consists of brushing the nails twice a day with an antiseptic soap starting 2 days before surgery. Antibiotic prophylaxis has to be discussed with patients affected by heart problems, particularly artificial heart valves, and joint prostheses.

Preoperative: A strict aseptic technique is necessary.

Postoperative: If infection is suspected, bacteriological lab tests should be carried out. Staphylococcus-fast antibiotics are given until the results of bacterial culture and sensitivity testing are available to avoid (methicillin-resistant) *Staphylococcus aureus* (MRSA).

Appearance of a greenish hue of the nail plate suggests a *Pseudomonas* infection and one should look for osteomyelitis radiologically. However, any greenish nail should not be operated until sufficiently treated; digit baths with diluted vinegar or bleach are usually effective.

Ischemia, Necrosis

2–3 mL should be enough for anesthesia of the digit. Higher volume may interfere with the vascularization by leading to a garrotte effect. If the surgery will take a longer period, the tourniquet should be opened every 20 min.

Even without overt infection, necrosis may be seen when sutures are too tight and/or not removed in time, or when swelling occurs after surgery and stays for a long time. Necrosis of the digit when the tourniquet has been left in place was repeatedly observed.

Recurrences

Recurrences depend on the nature of the original lesion and the type and extent of surgery. It is the worst complication in surgery of malignant tumors.

Temporary Abnormalities

- *Longitudinal nail fissure* can occur after matrix scarring of up to 3 mm.
- *Pseudo hernia of the matrix:* Loss or reduction of the overlying nail plate can result in a temporary tumid matrix bulging above the nail bed.

Permanent Residual Defects

These lead to unsightly scarring.

- *Crush injury:* This type of injury may lead to disruption of matrix and nail bed into small pieces. If these fragments are not meticulously incorporated into the repair, some may grow independently, cause implantation cysts, nail horns or spicules, and traumatic nail dystrophy.
- *Dorsal pterygium*: This type of pterygium develops when a scar bridges the undersurface of the proximal nail fold with the matrix and nail bed thus obscuring the cul-de-sac. Repositioning the nail plate into the cul-de-sac usually avoids this complication. If the width of the dorsal pterygium is small, repair may be attempted: The proximal nail fold fusion is separated from the matrix and the scar is excised and sutured with 6-0 absorbable sutures. The ventral surface of the proximal nail fold is grafted with a split-thickness nail bed graft (Shepard 1990). Finally, a nail plate substitute is inserted into the cul-de-sac to prevent that the roof and the bottom of the nail pocket can grow together again.
- For operations involving the lunula border, it is cosmetically important to maintain the curvilinear configuration of the distal lunula, which plays an important role in shaping the free edge of the nail plate.
- *Onycholysis* can occur after removal of tumors of the phalanx or when the nail bed is widely scarred. In severe cases, a split thickness nail bed graft taken from the big toe may be effective.
- *Ventral pterygium*: Hyponychial interventions may leave a painful ventral pterygium. If a topical treatment with hydroxychitosan fails, there are two surgical options: a strip of nail bed and hyponychium is resected and replaced by a split-thickness skin graft, or the ventral pterygium is removed by electrosection and a silicone strip is inserted to prevent early re-attachment of the pulp skin to the nail bed.
- *Nail deformities* have occurred after subungual hematoma, particularly if not released by drilling the nail plate, and from rough or careless avulsion of the nail to expose the bed. Nail deformities may also occur from the use of vicryl sutures in nail bed repair. These sutures, if too large, dissolve too slowly and are still present during the new nail growth. This can temporarily produce an area of onycholysis and ridging in the nail.
- *Longitudinal erythronychia* or *leukonychia* may be secondary and result from any matrix and nail bed scarring.
- *Longitudinal nail fissure* may be persistent if there is a longitudinal scar in the matrix or a small scar with a diameter wider than 3 mm, or secondary to median longitudinal nail unit excision.
- *Lateral deviation* of the nail plate may follow lateral longitudinal biopsy wider than 3 mm. CO_2 laser vaporization for periungual warts has produced the same abnormality.

Unpredictable Complications

Hypertrophic scar and *keloid* may involve the proximal nail fold and the nail bed. Intralesional steroid, methotrexate or bleomycin injections associated with silicone gel and/or sheets may be effective.

Reflex sympathetic dystrophy, now better known as *"Complex regional pain syndrome* (CRPS)*"* rarely occurs after nail surgery (Shepard 1990; Bussa et al. 2015). It presents with pain, sensitivity, and motor disturbances, along with autonomic nerve and even soft tissue trophic changes. Nail changes reported in the setting of CRPS include decrease of linear nail growth, Beau's line, onychomadesis, leukonychia, trachyonychia, brittleness, nail overcurvature, paronychia, and clubbing. Toes are usually spared.

CRPS Type I is mainly distinguished from Type II by not having demonstrable large nerve surgery. CRPS is more common in the upper extremity in women between 50 and 60. As there are no specific tests available, diagnosis is made using the "Budapest clinical criteria."

Epidermoid inclusion cyst may appear in a surgical scar. This lesion is not uncommon as a complication of inadequate surgery for ingrowing toenails.

Nail spicules are very common after wedge excisions for ingrown nails, but also develop after insufficient lateral matricectomies, lateral longitudinal excisions, or total nail apparatus removal. Postphenol nail spicules are most often seen in the first 3 months after the surgery in the proximal nail groove or in the middle of the proximal nail fold.

Nail Deformity

Damage of the matrix will lead to disturbance in nail formation. Circumscribed matrix injury, such as a longitudinal scar, leads to a furrow or split; hence matrix surgeries should, whenever possible, be oriented transversely. More severe nail injury causes a defective nail.

Nail bed injury with scarring leads to onycholysis; the more distal the scar the more obvious is the onycholysis. Large onycholysis of the big toenail results in loss of counterpressure of the nail plate to the distal nail bed during gait with resultant distal bulge formation and shrinkage of the nail bed, called "disappearing nail bed." The nail cannot overgrow the distal bulge and becomes thicker, opaque, and yellow. Over time, the distal dorsal tuft of the bone is pulled upwards making conservative treatment ineffective.

Granulation Tissue

Granulation tissue usually develops on an open wound and is identical with phase two of wound healing. However, when a wound is not re-epithelializing in a certain time period or a wound is caused, and kept open, by a foreign body like an ingrown nail, granulation tissue often develops as a protruding tumor and may be mistaken for a pyogenic granuloma. However, the latter is, in fact, an eruptive lobular angioma and must not be confused with granulation tissue. Though the granulation tissue always grows bacteria on its surface it is not infectious in nature and does not respond to antibiotics although these may temporarily reduce its size and associated pain of perilesional inflammation.

Specific Complications

Some complications may be observed in any type of nail surgery (Table 23.2).

Cryosurgery

Complications of cryosurgery may be (Heidenheim and Jemec 1991):

Immediate

Pain, hemorrhage and necrosis, edema, blister formation, syncope (indirect)

Delayed

Postoperative infection, granulation tissue formation, dystrophy, leukonychia, distal nerve lesions (dysesthesia).

Prolonged

Hyper or hypopigmentation, atrophy, anonychia (usually transient)

TABLE 23.2

Possible Surgical Complications

Type of surgery	Possible complications
Proximal matrix punch biopsy >3 mm	Nail plate splitting
Distal matrix biopsy (transversally oriented)	Thinning of the nail plate
Nail bed biopsy (vertically oriented)	If > 4 mm: Onycholysis
Lateral-longitudinal biopsy	Lateral nail deviation
	Narrowing of the nail
	Spicule in case of persistence of the lateral horn of the matrix
Total nail avulsion	Nail thickening
	Overcurvature
	Anterior embedding
Partial matricectomy with surgical blade	Spicule, narrow nail, recurrence, onychomadesis
Partial matricectomy with phenol	Narrow nail
	Spicule
	Onycholysis, onychomadesis
	Perionychial burn
	Periostitis
	Recurrence
Procedure involving the proximal nail fold	Extensor tendon wound
	DIP (Distal interphalangeal) arthritis
	Joint pain
	Dorsal pterygium
	Dystrophy
	Hypertrophic scar
Fish mouth soft tissue surgery	Necrosis
CO_2 laser for periungual warts	Dystrophy
	Lateral deviation of the nail plate
En bloc ablation of the nail apparatus	Spicule
	Functional trouble of the finger
Skin grafting	Necrosis
	Implantation cyst
Cryosurgery	See Table 23.3

TABLE 23.3

Conditions Precluding Cryosurgery Use

Agammaglobulinemia	Cryofibrinogenemia
Blood dyscrasies of unknown origin	Cryoglobulinemia
Cold intolerance	Lupus pernio
Cold urticaria	Multiple myeloma
Collagen and autoimmune disease	Platelet deficiency disease
Concurrent immunosuppressive drugs	Pyoderma gangrenosum
Concurrent treatment with renal dialysis	Raynaud's disease

Source: See further Zacharian 1996.

Occupational (Belhadjali et al. 2006)

Numbness of the tip of the right index finger and the thumb has been noted as a side effect of cryo-therapy in the treating physician. It would seem that even brief contact with the nitrogen-cold nozzle or a cryosurgical unit is sufficient to induce superficial neural damage in the fingertips provided that exposure occurs repeatedly. Interestingly, workers dealing with frozen shrimps may also experience nail dystrophy and paronychia.

Many concurrent diseases should in general preclude the use of cryosurgery, they were listed by Zacarian (1986).

BIBLIOGRAPHY

Belhadjali H., Hanchi A., Chaari N. et al. (2006) Les dermatoses professionnelles chez les ouvriers de congélation et de conditionnement des produits de la mer de la région de Mahdia (Tunisie). *Ann Dermatol Venereol*; 133: 4S 283.

Bussa M., Guttilla D., Lucia M., Mascara A. et al. (2015) Complex regional pain syndrome type I: a comprehensive review. *Acta Anaesthesiol Scand*; 59: 685–697.

Clark A., Jellinek N. J. (2016) Intralesional injection for inflammatory nail diseases. *Dermatol Surg*; 42: 257–260.

Connolly K. L., Nehal K. S., Dusza S. W., Rossi A. M., Lee E. H. (2016) Assessment of intraoperative pain during Mohs micrographic surgery (MMS): an opportunity for improved patient care. *J Am Acad Dermatol*; 75: 590–594.

Cox C., Yao J. (2012) Tourniquet usage in upper extremity surgery. *J Hand Surg Am*; 35:1360–1361.

Guerrero-Gonzales G. A., Di Chiacchio N. G., D'Apparecida Machado-Filho C. (2016) Complex regional pain syndrome after nail surgery. *Dermatol Surg*; 42: 1116–1118.

Heidenheim M., Jemec G. B. (1991) Side-effects of cryotherapy. *J Am Acad Dermatol*; 24: 653.

Howe N., Cherpelis B. (2013) Obtaining rapid and effective hemostasis. Part I. Update and review of topical hemostatic agents. *J Am Acad Dermatol*; 69: 659–675.

Shepard G. H. (1990) Nail grafts for reconstruction. *Hand Clin*; 6:79–102 (discussion103).

Zacarian S. A. (1986) *Cryosurgery for skin cancer and cutaneous disorders*. CV Mosby Co, St Louis, USA, 283–297.

24

The painful nail

Robert Baran
Eckart Haneke

Painful nail is a frequent condition. The sensory nerves to the dorsum of the distal phalanges of the second, third, and fourth fingers are derived from fine oblique branches of the volar collateral nerves. Longitudinal branches of the dorsal collateral nerves supply the nails of the thumb and the fifth digit. The dorsal branches usually run to the nail fold and pass under the nail bed at the level of the lunula, although there are minor variations.

The distal digit has sensory and autonomic nerves. Autonomic nerves are nonmyelinated and end in fine arborizations. Sensory nerves end in either free nerve endings or special end-organ receptors. Pain and temperature are perceived by a dermal network of unmyelinated free nerve endings. Special receptors include abundant Merkel-Ranvier endings, Meissner's corpuscles, and Vater-Pacini corpuscles. Merkel's endings are touch receptors that associate with basal cells in the deep aspect of intermediate rete ridges, and they also are generally found elsewhere in the skin. In contrast, Meissner's and Vater-Pacini corpuscles are associated especially in the distal digit, although they are not unique to this site (Morgan et al., 2001).

For causes of pain see Table 24.1.

TABLE 24.1

Main Causes (see further Fiona A, Richert B. Onychalgia. *SAD* 2020; 6: 77–87).

Trauma	Foreign body
	Subungual hematoma
	Distal phalanx fracture
	Repeated microtrauma (shoes)
Inflammatory	Acute paronychia, herpes simplex
	Ingrown nails, pincer nails
	Osteitis, ventral pterygium
	Digital sarcoidosis
	Drugs, lupus erythematosus
Tumors	Glomus tumor, subungual leiomyoma, subungual corn
	Keratoacanthoma, subungual keratosis of incontinentia pigmenti
	Exostosis, osteochondroma, osteoid osteoma
	Subungual myxoid cyst, foreign body
	Epidermal implantation cyst
Vascular	Chilblain, Ice
	Raynaud's disease
	Systemic scleroderma, acrosclerosis
	Reflex sympathetic dystrophy (complex regional pain syndrome)

BIBLIOGRAPHY

Fiona A, Richert B (2020) Onychalgia. *Skin Appendage Disord*; 6:77–87.

Morgan A, Baran R, Haneke E (2001) Anatomy of the Nail unit in relation to the distal digit. In: Krull EA, Zook EG, Baran R, Haneke E *Nail surgery. A Text and Atlas*, Lippincott, Williams and Wilkins.

25

Radiation and the nail

Robert Baran

Postirradiation

Longitudinal melanonychia has been well described post irradiation associated with psoralen plus ultraviolet A (PUVA), neoplasms, and several medications. Transverse melanonychia is uncommon (Baumert et al. 2015). It was reported in patients following radio therapy to treat hand dermatitis (Shelley et al. 2015), PUVA therapy in psoriasis (Kaptanoglu and Oskay 2014), infliximab and patients infected with HIV were more likely to have transverse lines in their nails. Finally, these lines can be secondary to total skin electron beam therapy 2 to 4 months after patients were started on treatment (Quinlan et al. 2005). One case acquired, apparent and transient total leukonychia was also observed in association with total skin electron beam irradiation (Eros et al. 2011). Usually, dystrophic nails are observed.

Nail radiodermatitis

Nail involvement makes up one of the pathognomonic and early lesions of chronic hand radiodermatitis. These radiolesions sparing the thumbs involved especially the members of occupations – pediatricians, surgeons, engineers, etc. – who used radiology for a prolonger period. As an epidermicidal dose is reached, the skin appendages progressively appear atrophic and disappear. Then, there is a consistantly a benign lesion of vascular origin, "coal spots" that are very small dark punctate spots located in the upper part of the dermis of the nail bed, consequently visible by transparency beneath the nail and made of heaps of hemosiderin.

The nail matrix produces a longitudinally ridged and more or less dystrophic nail plate.

The second state presents with keratosis and atrophic skin with telangiectasia surrounding the dorsum of the plate. The latter becomes brownish, thickened, or thin with fissures of the free edge. Sometimes, the nail becomes opaque and brittle with koilonychia, or on the contrary with onychogryposis. The free edge can be elevated by a subungual wart. Those warts are sometimes annoying and even painful. The coal spots follow the extremely slow nail growth and may appear as longitudinal melanonychia. Paronychial infection is a painful complication, inflammatory or more often suppurating, or associated with dermatitis of the dorsal aspect of the terminal phalanx. Finally, infection reaches the subungual area, which becomes very painful. It can lead to nail avulsion which reveals an atonic ulceration.

The choice of treatment depends on the stage of the radiodermatitis:

- At the first stage of epidermal radiodermatitis with discrete longitudinal ridging and minute "coal spots," the lesions are likely to settle down.
- At the second stage, excision of atrophic skin and keratosis, followed by free grafting should be done.

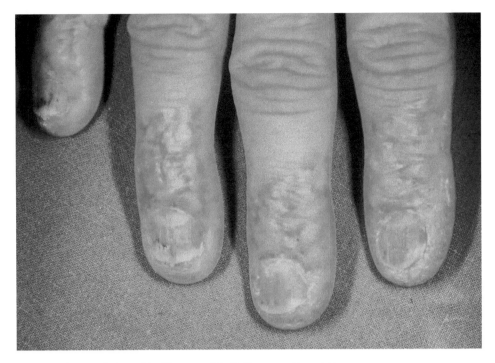

FIGURE 25.1   Acute radiodermatitis. (Courtesy of Dr S. Goettmann-Bonvalot.)

- As time passes, malignant transformation is almost unavoidable. If the cancer does not start often beneath the nail this area is nevertheless often invaded by the adjacent infiltrating tumor.

Soft radiotherapy evidently resulted in extensive transverse nail pigmentation affecting the treated fingers. However, we have observed a case of acute radiodermatitis on follow-up of an unexpected machine defect involving all the psoriatic fingernails of the patient (Figure 25.1).

Microwave radiation can cause transverse ridging, onycholysis and other plate dystrophies.

Brodkin and Bleiberg (1973) reported nil damage in restaurant workers exposed to a faulty microwave oven. They emphasized that the nail matrix may be damaged by microwave-induced thermal injury without the sensation of heat being felt by the oven user.

BIBLIOGRAPHY

Baumert B. G., Wodarski C., Klein C. et al. (2015) *Radiother ONCOL*; 114: 282–283.

Brodkin R. H., Bleiberg J. (1973) Cutaneous microwave injury. Report of two cases. *Acta Dermato-Venereol*; 53: 50–52.

Erös N., Marschaldo M., Bajcsay A. et al. (2011) Transient leukonychia after total skin electron beam irradiation. *JEADV*; 25: 115–116.

Kaptanoglu A. F., Oskay T. (2014) Symmetrical melanonychia of the thumbnails associated with PUVA in psoriasis. *J Dermatol*; 31: 148–150.

Quinlan K. E., Janiga J. J., Baran R. et al. (2005) Transverse melanonychia secondary to total skin electron beam therapy. A report of 3 cases. *JAAD*; 53: S 112–S 114.

Shelley W. B., Rawnsley H.M. Pillsbury D.M. (2015) *Radiother Oncol*; 114: 282-.

Index

Note: *Italicized* page numbers refer to figures, **bold** page numbers refer to tables

For Product Safety Concerns and Information please contact our EU representative GPSR@taylorandfrancis.com Taylor & Francis Verlag GmbH, Kaufingerstraße 24, 80331 München, Germany

T - #0175 - 090625 - C200 - 254/178/9 - PB - 9780367334789 - Gloss Lamination